Neuromonitoring and Assessment

Editor

CATHERINE HARRIS

CRITICAL CARE NURSING CLINICS OF NORTH AMERICA

www.ccnursing.theclinics.com

Consulting Editor
JAN FOSTER

March 2016 • Volume 28 • Number 1

ELSEVIER

1600 John F. Kennedy Boulevard • Suite 1800 • Philadelphia, Pennsylvania, 19103-2899

http://www.theclinics.com

CRITICAL CARE NURSING CLINICS OF NORTH AMERICA Volume 28, Number 1
March 2016 ISSN 0899-5885, ISBN-13: 978-0-323-41643-6

Editor: Kerry Holland
Developmental Editor: Colleen Viola

Critical Care Nursing Clinics of North America (ISSN 0899-5885) is published quarterly by Elsevier Inc., 360 Park Avenue South, New York, NY 10010-1710. Months of issue are March, June, September, and December. Business and Editorial Offices: 1600 John F. Kennedy Blvd., Suite 1800, Philadelphia, PA 19103-2899. Periodicals postage paid at New York, NY and additional mailing offices. Subscription prices are $155.00 per year for US individuals, $370.00 per year for US institutions, $100.00 per year for US students and residents, $200.00 per year for Canadian individuals, $464.00 per year for Canadian institutions, $230.00 per year for international individuals, $464.00 per year for international institutions and $115.00 per year for Canadian and international students/residents. To receive student/resident rate, orders must be accompanied by name of affiliated institution, data of term, and the *signature* of program/residency coordinator on institution letterhead. Orders will be billed at individual rate until proof of status is received. Foreign air speed delivery is included in all *Clinics* subscription prices. All prices are subject to change without notice. **POSTMASTER:** Send address changes to *Critical Care Nursing Clinics of North America*, Elsevier Health Sciences Division, Subscription Customer Service, 3251 Riverport Lane, Maryland Heights, MO 63043. **Customer Service: 1-800-654-2452 (US and Canada); 314-447-8871 (outside US and Canada). Fax: 314-447-8029. E-mail:** JournalsCustomerService-usa@elsevier.com **(for print support) and** JournalsOnlineSupport-usa@elsevier.com **(for online support).**

Reprints. For copies of 100 or more of articles in this publication, please contact the Commercial Reprints Department, Elsevier Inc., 360 Park Avenue South, New York, New York, 10010-1710; Tel.: 212-633-3874, Fax: 212-633-3820, and E-mail: reprints@elsevier.com.

Critical Care Nursing Clinics of North America is covered in *MEDLINE/PubMed (Index Medicus), International Nursing Index, Nursing Citation Index, Cumulative Index to Nursing and Allied Health Literature, and RNdex Top 100.*

Contributors

CONSULTING EDITOR

JAN FOSTER, PhD, APRN, CNS
Formerly, Associate Professor, College of Nursing, Texas Woman's University, Houston; Currently, President, Nursing Inquiry and Intervention Inc., The Woodlands, Texas

EDITOR

CATHERINE HARRIS, PhD, MBA, AGACNP, ANP, FNP-BC
Assistant Professor, Graduate Programs; Director, Adult Gerontology Acute Care Nurse Practitioner Program, Jefferson College of Nursing; Nurse Practitioner, Neurocritical Care, Jefferson Hospital for Neuroscience, Philadelphia, Pennsylvania

AUTHORS

OLIVIA AMENDOLIA, BA, BSN, RN
Department of Nursing, Hospital of the University of Pennsylvania, Philadelphia, Pennsylvania

RAMANI BALU, MD, PhD
Department of Neurology, University of Pennsylvania, Philadelphia, Pennsylvania

BRITTANY BECKMANN, BSN, RN
Department of Nursing, Hospital of the University of Pennsylvania, Philadelphia, Pennsylvania

KATHRYN BURKE, BSN, RN
Penn Presbyterian Medical Center, Philadelphia, Pennsylvania

LAUREN CIOCCO, BSN, RN
Department of Nursing, Hospital of the University of Pennsylvania, Philadelphia, Pennsylvania

MARIAN FEIL, DNP, CRNA, MSN
Thomas Jefferson University, Philadelphia, Pennsylvania

MEGAN FISHEL, RN, BSN, CCRN
The University of Texas Southwestern, Dallas, Texas

SUZANNE FRANGOS, RN, CNRN
Department of Neurosurgery, University of Pennsylvania, Philadelphia, Pennsylvania

JOSEPH B. HAYMORE, MS, ACNP-BC, CRNP
Senior Nurse Practitioner, Neurocritical Care Unit, University of Maryland Medical Center; Doctor of Nursing Practice Student, University of Maryland School of Nursing, Baltimore, Maryland

CAREY HECK, PhD, CRNP, ACNP-BC, CCRN, CNRN
Assistant Professor, College of Nursing, Thomas Jefferson University, Philadelphia, Pennsylvania

CHRISTOPHER HYLKEMA, MSN, RN, CEN, CFRN
Thomas Jefferson University Hospital, Thomas Jefferson University, Philadelphia, Pennsylvania

NICOLE A. IRICK, RN, BSN, CCRN
Thomas Jefferson University, Philadelphia, Pennsylvania

ATUL KALANURIA, MD, FACP
Department of Neurology, University of Pennsylvania, Philadelphia, Pennsylvania

JAY KOREN, BSN, RN
Nurse Manager, Surgical Intensive Care Unit, The MetroHealth System, Cleveland, Ohio

MONISHA KUMAR, MD
Department of Neurology, Perelman School of Medicine, University of Pennsylvania, Philadelphia, Pennsylvania

SARAH L. LIVESAY, DNP, RN, APRN
Associate Professor, Department of Adult and Gerontology Health, Rush University College of Nursing, Chicago, Illinois

EILEEN MALONEY-WILENSKY, MSN, ACNP-BC
Department of Neurosurgery, University of Pennsylvania, Philadelphia, Pennsylvania

BETHANN MARION, BSN, RN
Department of Nursing, Hospital of the University of Pennsylvania, Philadelphia, Pennsylvania

MOLLY McNETT, PhD, RN, CNRN
Director, Nursing Research, The MetroHealth System, Cleveland, Ohio

KYLE McNULTY
Department of Nursing, Hospital of the University of Pennsylvania, Philadelphia, Pennsylvania

KIMBERLY MILLER, BSN, RN
Department of Nursing, Hospital of the University of Pennsylvania, Philadelphia, Pennsylvania

DAIWAI M. OLSON, RN, PhD, CCRN, FNCS
The University of Texas Southwestern, Dallas, Texas

NIKHIL PATEL, MD, MBA
Resident, Department of Neurology, University of Maryland School of Medicine, Baltimore, Maryland

AMY DELLA PENNA, MSN, RN, CCRN
Clinical Specialist, Neuroscience Intensive Care Unit, Thomas Jefferson University Hospital, Philadelphia, Pennsylvania

JENNIFER D. ROBINSON, MS, APRN, RN, CNRN
Neurocritical Care Nurse Practitioner, Lead Neuroscience Quality & Safety Practitioner, Yale New Haven Hospital, New Haven, Connecticut

DONNAMARIE SCHUELE, BSN, RN
Department of Nursing, Hospital of the University of Pennsylvania, Philadelphia, Pennsylvania

MARIE WILSON, MSN, RN, CRNP, CCRN, CNRN
Nurse Manager, Neuroscience Intensive Care Unit, Thomas Jefferson University Hospital, Philadelphia, Pennsylvania

DANIELLE WRIGHT, BSN, RN
Department of Nursing, Hospital of the University of Pennsylvania, Philadelphia, Pennsylvania

SUSAN YEAGER, MS, RN, CCRN, ACNP-BC, FNCS
Neurocritical Care Lead Nurse Practitioner, The Ohio State University Wexner Medical Center; Clinical Instructor, College of Nursing, The Ohio State University, Columbus, Ohio

BETHANY YOUNG, MSN, RN, AGCNS-BC
Department of Nursing, Hospital of the University of Pennsylvania, Philadelphia, Pennsylvania

Contents

> Although technology over the past several decades has enabled improved neuroimaging and advanced noninvasive and invasive neuromonitoring, the role of the bedside nurse conducting ongoing neurologic examination is still a foundational element of neuromonitoring. Ongoing neurologic monitoring by the bedside nurse in the neuroscience intensive care unit is variable and guided by little evidence or data. When neurologic monitoring through clinical examination is possible, data obtained from multimodal monitoring should be interpreted in the context of the neurologic examination. The bedside nurse plays a crucial role in conducting ongoing neurologic examinations.

> Blood pressure (BP) management is essential in neurocritical care settings to ensure adequate cerebral perfusion and prevent secondary brain injury. Despite consensus on the importance of BP monitoring, significant practice variations persist regarding optimal methods for monitoring and treatment of BP values among patients with neurologic injuries. This article provides a summary of research investigating various approaches for BP management in neurocritical care. Evidence-based recommendations, areas for future research, and current technological advancements for BP management are discussed.

> This article reviews current literature regarding the neuro intensive care unit (ICU) and the ICU setting in general regarding delirium, pain, agitation, and evidence-based guidelines and assessment tools. Delirium in the ICU affects as many as 50% to 80% of patients. Delirium is associated with increased burden of illness, higher mortality, and increased suffering. Evidence-based guidelines recommend using validated and reliable assessment tools. We reviewed current national clinical guidelines, validated tools for assessing pain, agitation/sedation, and delirium. We also reviewed a delirium risk-assessment/prediction tool.

Ultrasound has been used for almost 30 years in a wide variety of clinical applications and environments. From the austerity of battlefields to the labor and delivery ward, ultrasound has the ability to give clinicians real-time, noninvasive diagnostic imaging. Ultrasound by emergency physicians (and all nonradiologists) has become more prevalent and has been used for examinations such as the transcranial Doppler to evaluate for stroke, cardiac function, FAST and EFAST examinations for trauma, and now increased intracranial pressure (ICP) via Optic Nerve Sheath Diameter Ultrasound (ONSD). The ONSD is a valid and reliable indicator of ICP.

 Video content accompanies this article at http://www.ccnursing. theclinics.com/

The neurologic examination (neuroexamination) is one of the most powerful tools available to nurses and physicians caring for patients with neurologic or neurosurgical illness. Assessing cranial nerve function is one of the most vital components of the neuroexamination. The pupillary light reflex helps to evaluate the status of the second and third cranial nerves and is one of the most well-known elements of the cranial nerve examination. Automated pupillometers have been developed that provide objective measures of size of the pupil and the responsiveness of the pupil to light (neuropupillary index).

A variety of neuromonitoring techniques are available to aid in the care of neurocritically ill patients. However, traditional monitors lack the ability to measure brain biochemistry and may provide inadequate warning of potentially reversible deleterious conditions. Cerebral microdialysis (CMD) is a safe, novel method of monitoring regional brain biochemistry. Analysis of CMD analytes as part of a multimodal approach may help inform clinical decision-making, guide medical treatments, and aid in prognostication of patient outcome. Its use is most frequently documented in traumatic brain injury and subarachnoid hemorrhage. Incorporating CMD into clinical practice is a multidisciplinary effort.

There are many approaches to and opportunities for implementing temperature modulation in critically ill patients, but barriers also exist.

Conceptually, the process of cooling is rather straightforward; however, targeted temperature management is anything but simplistic. The need for a collaborative approach (physicians champions, nursing support, respiratory therapists, pharmacists, laboratory personnel, and supply chain representatives) to address definitions of normothermia and fever, patient inclusion/exclusion criteria for therapy based on underlying neurorelated pathologies, determination of methods of induction/maintenance, monitoring required, education planning, and strategies to minimize potential complications are warranted.

CRITICAL CARE NURSING
CLINICS OF NORTH AMERICA

THE CLINICS ARE AVAILABLE ONLINE!
Access your subscription at:
www.theclinics.com

Preface

Neuromonitoring in the Intensive Care Unit

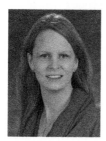

Catherine Harris, PhD, MBA, AGACNP, ANP, FNP-BC
Editor

This issue of *Critical Care Nursing Clinics of North America* is focused on neuromonitoring in the intensive care unit (ICU). Neuromonitoring is a broad umbrella term that elicits different concepts depending on a person's role in the ICU. For instance, a trauma nurse may associate neuromonitoring with intracranial bolts, whereas an ultrasound technician may immediately think of transcranial Dopplers. A neuro ICU nurse may have visions of going to multiple scans or working with external ventricular drains. The term neuromonitoring includes all these concepts as well as more, which are discussed within this dedicated issue of *Critical Care Nursing Clinics of North America*.

In designing this issue, we created three overriding themes of neuromonitoring that remained fairly broad. First, we thought of traditional methods of neuromonitoring that a nurse would expect to see in this issue. Robinson goes into depth on treating refractory increased intracranial pressures, while Heck discusses different modalities that are available for using invasive neuromonitoring for patients. Irick and Feil provide an extremely helpful overview of neuromonitoring in the operating room. Many ICU nurses are not familiar with neuromonitoring in the operating room, and the literature is resource-poor in this area. Therefore, the collaborative approach from Irick and Feil not only provides a better understanding of neuromonitoring but also gives nurses a glimpse into the role of the nurse anesthetist.

The second approach we took on neuromonitoring was to explore novel concepts and products. Hylkema provides a look at one of the newest concepts of using optic sheath ultrasound as a method for assessing intracranial pressures noninvasively. The use of ultrasound has grown exponentially over the years due to its ease of use, low cost, and accessibility. Hylkema provides an overview of how it is being used for neurologic patients. Few centers have microdialysis, but the road on how to use it is being mapped by Kumar and Young in this issue. Even if your hospital setting does not use microdialysis, there is tremendous value in understanding brain metabolism. Wilson and Della Penna present evidenced-based research on the value of

Crit Care Nurs Clin N Am 28 (2016) xiii–xiv
http://dx.doi.org/10.1016/j.cnc.2015.12.001
0899-5885/16/$ – see front matter © 2016 Published by Elsevier Inc.

thermoregulation in the neurologically impaired patients and treatment options. Olson and Fishel provide an astounding wealth of information on the value of pupillometry and how it can be used in the ICU.

We took some liberty in expanding the concept of neuromonitoring to encompass a nontraditional approach to the topic. Livesay highlights the fact that the nurse is indeed the most important part of the neuromonitoring armamentarium that we have. McNett reinforces that concept with the challenges nurses have with blood pressures in neuro patients. Why do we use mean arterial pressures? Haymore delves into his own research on delirium to show that nurses are the most important piece of the picture as their astuteness in evaluating changes, however subtle in patients, is essential. Finally, Yeager provides the most comprehensive review of neuroradiology that will likely remain as a resource for nurses for years to come!

We hope this issue of *Critical Care Nursing Clinics of North America* serves as a resource for ICU nurses who are seeking to better understand how to care for complex patients with a neurologic issue. The most important concept we want to convey in this issue is that no matter how much neurotechnology exists, the most critical neuro-monitoring process we have is the nurse. The nurse is the ultimate tool in neuromoni-toring. The nurse is the one who needs to understand, interpret, and troubleshoot the equipment. Without the knowledge and resourcefulness of the nurse, the technology can only provide output. The nurse's passion to improve care and outcomes in pa-tients with neurologic injury is pivotal, since no device can replace the care and pro-tective vigilance nursing brings to the table. Therefore, this special issue of Neuromonitoring is dedicated to the nurse in the ICU who is committed to working with patients with neurologic injuries and to improving his or her knowledge of what technology is out there.

Catherine Harris, PhD, MBA, AGACNP, ANP, FNP-BC
Adult Gerontology Acute Care Nurse Practitioner Program
Jefferson College of Nursing
Neurocritical Care, Jefferson Hospital for Neuroscience
901 Walnut Street, Suite 823
Philadelphia, PA 19107, USA

E-mail address:
Catherine.harris@jefferson.edu

The Bedside Nurse
The Foundation of Multimodal Neuromonitoring

Sarah L. Livesay, DNP, RN, APRN

KEYWORDS

- Neuroscience • Nursing • Assessment • Monitoring • Multimodal

KEY POINTS

- Monitoring of the patient's clinical neurologic examination is a fundamental role of the bedside nurse in the neuroscience intensive care unit.
- Few data exist to guide the content and frequency of ongoing neurologic monitoring.
- Data obtained through multimodal monitoring technology should be interpreted in the context of the neurologic examination obtained by the bedside nurse.
- Clinical scales are often used in ongoing neurologic monitoring. The scales used should be relevant to the patients' clinical status.
- Additional data are needed to guide when to stop frequent assessments and when frequent assessment may be associated with complications.

INTRODUCTION

Although technology over the past several decades has enabled improved neuroimaging and advanced noninvasive and invasive neuromonitoring, the role of the bedside nurse conducting ongoing neurologic examination is still a foundational element of neuromonitoring.[1] Eliciting a patient's history and conducting a physical examination are fundamental elements of medical and nursing care. When patients are in the neuroscience intensive care unit (NSICU), ongoing neurologic assessments are key to determining a patient's clinical status and response to interventions.

Despite the long-held notion that the nurse is the foundation of neuromonitoring, little evidence is available to guide the extent and frequency of neurologic monitoring in the NSICU. A complete, head-to-toe neurologic examination is both broad and time consuming. Ongoing neurologic assessment of patients in the NSICU usually consists of a focused neurologic examination tailored to a patient's diagnosis and illness

Relevant Disclosures: None.
Department of Adult and Gerontology Health, Rush University College of Nursing, 600 South Paulina Street, Chicago, IL 60612, USA
E-mail address: sarah_l_livesay@rush.edu

Crit Care Nurs Clin N Am 28 (2016) 1–8
http://dx.doi.org/10.1016/j.cnc.2015.10.002
0899-5885/16/$ – see front matter
ccnursing.theclinics.com

progression. However, few data exist to guide the content and frequency of the nurse's ongoing neurologic monitoring. Additionally, certain clinical conditions such as increased intracranial pressure render the patient unable to endure repeated stimulation through neurologic examination. Therefore, the bedside nurse must be astute in understanding both disease pathophysiology as well as the neurologic examination and how the examination findings localize to pathology in the brain. This review provides an overview of indications and state of the science for neurologic monitoring through clinical examination.

GOALS OF CLINICAL MONITORING THROUGH NEUROLOGIC ASSESSMENT

Patients with critical neurologic illness require intensive monitoring. The Consensus Summary Statement of the International Multidiscipline Consensus Conference on Multimodal Monitoring in Neurocritical Care (2014) provides an overview of the general goals of monitoring in this patient population (**Box 1**).[2] Specific to neurocritical care, ongoing monitoring of any kind should be aimed at detecting neurologic worsening, guiding patient care management, and individualizing decisions to the patient. When the nursing staff is deciding what to monitor and when, these goals are at forefront of tailoring the neurologic examination to the patient's needs. Although protocols and guidelines often guide care, the art of neurologic monitoring must be tailored to the patient.

The goals of monitoring outlined in the multimodal consensus document are similar to the goals published within nursing textbooks for decades. Nurses conduct a neurologic examination for a variety of reasons. Most broadly, a neurologic examination is conducted to determine if neurologic dysfunction exists, to determine the impact of existing dysfunction or impairment on patient's life, and to determine the overall neurologic impact of disease.[3] Ongoing clinical neurologic assessments in the NSICU specifically serve to establish a baseline for patient's clinical status, identifying whether deterioration is occurring and the severity of dysfunction, and monitor impact of interventions aimed at treating neurologic illness.[4] As other data are obtained through noninvasive and invasive techniques, they are interpreted in conjunction with the findings from the ongoing neurologic monitoring.

Box 1
Reasons to monitor patients with neurologic disorders who require critical care

Detect early neurologic worsening before irreversible brain damage occurs.

Individualize patient care decisions.

Guide patient management.

Monitor the physiologic response to treatment and avoid any adverse effects.

Allow clinical to better understand the pathophysiology of complex disorders.

Design and implement management protocols.

Improve neurologic outcome and quality of life in survivors of severe brain injury.

Through understanding disease pathophysiology, begin to develop new, mechanistically oriented therapies where treatments currently are lacking or are empiric in nature.

From Le Roux P, Menon DK, Citerio G, et al. Consensus summary statement of the International Multidisciplinary Consensus Conference on Multimodality Monitoring in Neurocritical Care: a statement for healthcare professionals from the Neurocritical Care Society and the European Society of Intensive Care Medicine. Intensive Care Med 2014;40(9):1189–209; with permission.

STATE OF THE SCIENCE: ONGOING NEUROLOGIC ASSESSMENT IN THE NEUROSCIENCE INTENSIVE CARE UNIT

Although clinical neurologic examination may be one of the most frequent tasks performed by the bedside nurse in the NSICU, little research or evidence exists to guide the frequency and content of the neurologic examination. Several publications suggest significant variability between inpatient programs regarding the content of ongoing neurologic assessments, as well as the timing and frequency of such assessments.[5] A lengthy neurologic examination is generally curtailed into a *neuro check* that is repeated frequently as a means of neuromonitoring. However, no standard approach to neuro checks exist and the essential components of the neuro check are often interpreted differently between organizations.

Even for the most fundamental components of neurologic assessment, trained clinicians may experience variability in interpreting assessment findings. Something as seemingly simple as pupil assessment is subject to variability between providers.[6] In a recent observational study, Olson and colleagues[7] found only moderate interrater reliability for pupil size and reactivity among more than 200 nurses and physicians. Therefore, an assessment activity as common as checking the pupil size and pupillary reflex is not as straightforward as previously thought. Such findings have helped to propel the use of technology such as digital pupillometers, a neurologic monitor, to help ensure consistency between caregivers. However, assessment findings from such technology are still placed in the context of the neurologic monitoring conducted by the bedside nurse.

According to the goals outlined, the neurologic assessment content, timing, and frequency should be dictated by the patient's neurologic illness and acuity, as well as management goals and interventions. However, many NSICUs use a combination of physician orders and unit standard practice to dictate the frequency and content of ongoing neurologic assessment and monitoring. Because there are no studies or clear guidelines to guide the standard practice in the NSICU, these guidelines should serve as a starting point from which the nurse and health care team may tailor monitoring to the needs of the patient.

National Clinical Practice Guidelines

National clinical practice guidelines vary in terms of the degree to which ongoing neurologic assessments are even addressed. The Neurocritical Care Society's Multimodal Monitoring Consensus Statement acknowledges the importance of clinical evaluation through assessment in multimodal monitoring.[8] Specifically, the consensus statement evaluated the role of coma assessment scales in patients with acute brain injury, as well as the role of pain assessment, sedation level assessment, and delirium assessment in this patient population. A summary of their recommendations is included in in **Box 2**. However, the guideline does not address ongoing neurologic monitoring further.

The American Stroke Association guidelines for the management of ischemic stroke, intracerebral hemorrhage, and subarachnoid hemorrhage are variable in how they address ongoing monitoring in the early management of these diseases. The most prescriptive guidance for tailoring the neurologic assessment according to these diagnoses is in patients who receive intravenous thrombolysis with recombinant activated tissue plasminogen activator. Because patients are at risk for neurologic deterioration from hemorrhagic conversion after recombinant activated tissue plasminogen activator administration, frequent neurologic assessment during the first 24 hours after recombinant activated tissue plasminogen activator administration is

---

Box 2

Summary of clinical evaluation recommendations from the consensus statement summary of the International Multidisciplinary Consensus Conference on Multimodal Monitoring in Neurocritical Care

1. Assessments with either the Glasgow Coma Score or Full Outline of Unresponsiveness score should be performed in comatose patients with acute brain injury (stroke recommendation, low quality of evidence).

2. Recommend using the numeric reporting scale to elicit the patient's self-report of pain in appropriate patients (stroke recommendation, low quality of evidence).

3. Recommend using behavior based scales to estimate pain in patients who are unable to self-report pain. Such scales may include the Behavioral Pain Scale or the Critical Care Pain Observation Tool (stroke recommendation, low quality of evidence).

4. Recommend the use of the Nociception Coma Scale—Revised to estimate pain for patients with severely impaired consciousness, such as a vegetative state or minimally conscious state (stroke recommendation, low quality of evidence).

5. Monitor sedation with a validated and reliable scale such as the Sedation–Agitation Scale or Richmond Agitation Sedation Scale (stroke recommendation, low quality of evidence).

Adapted from Le Roux P, Menon DK, Citerio G, et al. Consensus summary statement of the International Multidisciplinary Consensus Conference on Multimodality Monitoring in Neurocritical Care: a statement for healthcare professionals from the Neurocritical Care Society and the European Society of Intensive Care Medicine. Intensive Care Med 2014;40(9):1189–209; with permission.

---

supported by the American Stroke Association guidelines. Neurologic assessments should be conducted every 15 minutes for the first 2 hours, every 30 minutes for the next 6 hours, and then hourly for the remaining 16 hours.[9] These assessment criteria were based on the original trial evaluating the use of intravenous tissue plasminogen activator for ischemic stroke. Although it is logical that patients need intensive neurologic monitoring after thrombolysis because they are at risk for hemorrhage, no studies have evaluated the necessary frequency and duration of these assessments. A current clinical trial aims to examine the safety of a less frequent assessment scheme for patients with a lower stroke scale.[10]

Regardless of the thrombolysis status, the Comprehensive Overview of Nursing and Interdisciplinary Care of the Ischemic Stroke Patient guideline suggests that any patient admitted to the intensive care unit should undergo neurologic evaluation at least hourly and more frequently if necessary.[11] The guidelines also acknowledge that the National Institutes of Health Stroke Scale (NIHSS) may be a useful tool for initial and ongoing neurologic assessment in patients with ischemic stroke. However, neither recommendation was based on strong evidence.

The latest guidelines for the management of patients with intracerebral hemorrhage acknowledge that initial care should take place in the intensive care unit or dedicated stroke unit with a physician and nursing team who have neuroscience expertise.[12] Patients with intracerebral hemorrhage are at risk for neurologic deterioration and may require monitoring of intracranial pressure, cerebral perfusion pressure, and other physiologic parameters. The latest American Stroke Association guideline for the management of patients with subarachnoid hemorrhage does not address ongoing neurologic monitoring or nursing care.[13]

The latest guideline from the Brain Trauma Foundation on care of the patient with traumatic brain injury (TBI) does not address nursing monitoring through ongoing assessment.[14] However, the National Collaborating Center for Acute Care in the United Kingdom advocates for frequent monitoring of patients with head injury, and outlines minimum criteria to be included in neurologic assessment.[15] The group recommends that patients undergoing in-hospital neurologic monitoring for head injury should undergo neurologic observations that include the Glasgow Coma Scale (GCS), pupil size and reactivity, and limb movement along with other physiologic monitoring such as blood pressure, heart rate, blood oxygen saturation, and respiratory rate. They further state that on hospital admission, this assessment should occur every 30 minutes for 2 hours, every hour for 4 hours, and then every 2 hours thereafter. If the patient declines clinically at any time, neurologic observations should be conducted at least every 30 minutes. All recommendations were based on a low level of evidence.[15]

Clinical Monitoring and Outcomes

Although it is difficult to glean practice standards for ongoing neurologic assessment in critically ill patients with neurologic disease from national clinical practice guidelines, the importance of ongoing neurologic assessment by the bedside nursing and medical staff remains a key element of nursing care in an NSICU and a foundational element for neuromonitoring.[1] No studies have linked clinical monitoring with improved patient outcomes. However, trials have clearly associated care from a dedicated team with improved outcomes. Patients with stroke who receive care on a dedicated stroke unit have better outcomes, including a higher likelihood of surviving their stroke, as well as becoming independent.[16] Receiving care in an NSICU is generally associated with decreased mortality, improved quality metrics, and a lesser duration of stay.[17] This link between consistent and expert caregiver teams and improved patient outcomes is likely related at least in part to the knowledge and expertise of the nursing staff dedicated to a specific population. The improved outcomes may be at least partially attributed to the ongoing neurologic monitoring administered by the nursing staff. However, the studies on improved outcomes when like patients are grouped in one unit do not explore this relationship specifically.

Few studies are available to guide the frequency and necessary components of the neurologic examination during care in the neurocritical care unit. The lack of consensus on what to monitor and how frequently may contribute to confusion and variability in neurocritical care units across the nation. Despite this variability, there is evidence that limiting the components of the neurologic examination in patients with acute ischemic stroke is associated with missed assessment findings indicative of patient decline. The role of the NIHSS in the ongoing neurologic monitoring of patients with stroke has been somewhat controversial.[18] A number of modified or slim stroke scales have been validated for use in the care of patients with stroke. However, the ongoing monitoring of patients with stroke using the GCS or modified stroke scales as opposed to a full NIHSS may result in missing assessment findings indicative of critical neurologic decline. In a retrospective review of 172 patients with stroke, monitoring with GCS alone or modified stroke scales resulted in false-negative assessment findings in anywhere from 5% to 56% of cases, depending on which scale was used.[18] This suggests that a paired-down neurologic assessment may result in missed clinical changes that could signify neurologic worsening.

Clinical Monitoring and Adverse Outcomes

Frequent neurologic monitoring during acute neurologic illness may be critical to identifying neurologic decline. However, ongoing hourly neurologic assessment has the potential to disrupt crucial sleep rhythms, particularly over long ICU stays. One retrospective review of 124 patients with ICU admissions for TBI evaluated the length of hourly neurologic assessment and the likelihood of neurologic decline.[19] More than 70% of patients received hourly neurologic assessments on admission and for an average duration of 67.7 hours in this single-center report. Additionally, 18 of 124 patients received hourly neurologic assessments for longer than 4 days. The patients who received hourly assessment for longer than 4 days had a significantly longer duration of stay than the overall group, regardless of the severity of their TBI. Of the entire cohort of 124 patients, only 2 required neurosurgical intervention beyond 48 hours after their admission. This observational study suggests that prolonged hourly assessment may be associated with increased duration of stay, and may not be indicated routinely in patients with head injury beyond 48 hours without additional indication for monitoring, such as increased intracranial pressure or cerebral edema. The authors suggested a modified assessment schedule for stable patients with nonpenetrating head injury without large-volume hemorrhage, mass lesion, or midline shift and outlined plans to study this assessment schedule prospectively.[19]

Although the report from Stone and colleagues[19] is only 1 single center experience and included only patients with TBI, it calls into question the routine application of hourly neurologic assessments when patients are admitted to the neurologic ICU. Hourly assessments disrupt sleep–wake cycles and are associated with higher levels of circulating stress hormones.[20] Frequent assessments are critical when the patient is at high risk for decline, but frequent monitoring when it is no longer necessary may be detrimental to recovery.

Certain patient conditions may place them at increased risk for deterioration with repeated stimulation from a full neurologic examination, such as patients with an increased intracranial pressure. In such situations, multimodal neuromonitoring is essential to add crucial data about the patient's neurologic status. However, when a patient has a clinical examination to follow, data from multimodal monitoring should be interpreted in the context of the neurologic examination. However, additional research is needed to better guide the frequency and duration of ongoing neurologic monitoring for patients in the NSICU.

NEUROLOGIC MONITORING ASSESSMENT SCALES

A number of scales are available to the bedside nurse to use when conducting ongoing neurologic examinations. This includes scales to assess disordered consciousness such as the GCS and the Full Outline of Unresponsiveness Score, as well as assessment tools such as the NIHSS discussed elsewhere in this article. Although these tools are helpful to quantify deficits and quickly communicate patient status between caregivers, they should be applied with a degree of caution when used by the nurse for ongoing clinical monitoring. Most tools routinely used for ongoing neurologic monitoring were never developed with that intent. Even the GCS, which is used frequently to monitor the clinical status of patients in the NSICU, was never intended to be a sole indicator of neurologic status or clinical monitoring.[21] The GCS was intended to help quantify consciousness and to be used in conjunction with the rest of the neurologic examination.

As another example, the NIHSS has spread to be used routinely by bedside staff to monitor patients with all types of stroke. However, the NIHSS was originally developed to help quantify neurologic deficit from ischemic stroke to determine eligibility for acute treatment trials. The NIHSS associates a numeric value with a reasonably in-depth neurologic examination. However, the scale is less useful for patients with certain stroke syndromes, such as posterior circulation stroke, and patients with low scores may still experience significant neurologic deficit.[22] Therefore, the NIHSS should not be the only component of neurologic examination for all patients with stroke. Furthermore, no data exist that demonstrating how frequently the scale should be applied as a tool for ongoing clinical monitoring or in patients with intracerebral hemorrhage or subarachnoid hemorrhage. Scales should be assessed in light of the patient's condition to determine whether additional assessment components are necessary to best identify if the patient were to deteriorate clinically.

ROLE OF THE CLINICAL EXAMINATION IN MULTIMODAL NEUROMONITORING

As technology allows for multiple modes of monitoring patients, the clinical examination remains paramount to synthesize the data from monitors into meaningful information. Findings from advanced neurologic imaging, monitoring of intracranial pressure, brain tissue oxygenation, and other technology still must be placed in the context of patient progression. In situations where the neurologic examination is obscured by coma or by intervention such as sedation, multimodal monitoring is crucial to quantify neurologic status. In situations where a clinical examination is obtainable, multimodal monitoring should be interpreted in conjunction with the findings from the nurse's neurologic monitoring. Clinical assessment of consciousness and neurologic deficit helps to define the patient's progression and allows the team to make sense of the data from monitoring and to tailor interventions accordingly.

SUMMARY

The bedside nurse plays a fundamental role in neuromonitoring through ongoing clinical examination of the patient. However, the nuances of what should be assessed and how frequently remains poorly studied. Routine frequencies and the use of scales may be helpful to ensure consistency, but may result in missing key findings relevant to the patient's situation, and may be detrimental in certain clinical situations. Additional studies are needed to better define the role of neurologic examination in the routine care of patients in the NSICU. When neurologic monitoring by the bedside nurse is possible, it serves as the foundation of interpreting additional data obtained through multimodal monitoring.

REFERENCES

1. Stocchetti N, Le Roux P, Vespa P, et al. Clinical review: neuromonitoring - an update. Crit Care 2013;17(1):201.
2. Le Roux P, Menon DK, Citerio G, et al. Consensus summary statement of the international multidisciplinary consensus conference on multimodality monitoring in neurocritical care: a statement for healthcare professionals from the neurocritical care society and the European society of intensive care medicine. Neurocrit Care 2014;21(Suppl 2):S1–26.
3. Hickey JV. The clinical practice of neurological and neurosurgical nursing. 7th edition. 2013.
4. Iacono LA, Wells C, Mann-Finnerty K. Standardizing neurological assessments. J Neurosci Nurs 2014;46(2):125–32.
5. Gocan S, Fisher A. Neurological assessment by nurses using the National Institutes of Health Stroke Scale: implementation of best practice guidelines. Can J Neurosci Nurs 2008;30(3):31–42.
6. Clark A, Clarke TN, Gregson B, et al. Variability in pupil size estimation. Emerg Med J 2006;23(6):440–1.

7. Olson DM, Stutzman S, Saju C, et al. Interrater reliability of pupillary assessments. Neurocrit Care 2015. [Epub ahead of print].
8. Le Roux P, Menon DK, Citerio G, et al. Consensus summary statement of the international multidisciplinary consensus conference on multimodality monitoring in neurocritical care: a statement for healthcare professionals from the Neurocritical Care Society and the European Society of Intensive Care Medicine. Intensive Care Med 2014;40(9):1189–209.
9. Jauch EC, Saver JL, Adams HP Jr, et al. Guidelines for the early management of patients with acute ischemic stroke: a guideline for healthcare professionals from the American Heart Association/American Stroke Association. Stroke 2013;44(3): 870–947.
10. clinicaltrials.gov. Safety study of post intravenous tPA monitoring in ischemic stroke (OPTIMIST). 2015. Available at: https://clinicaltrials.gov/ct2/show/NCT02039375. Accessed September 14, 2015.
11. Summers D, Leonard A, Wentworth D, et al. Comprehensive overview of nursing and interdisciplinary care of the acute ischemic stroke patient: a scientific statement from the American Heart Association. Stroke 2009;40(8):2911–44.
12. Hemphill JC 3rd, Greenberg SM, Anderson CS, et al. Guidelines for the management of spontaneous intracerebral hemorrhage: a guideline for healthcare professionals from the American Heart Association/American Stroke Association. Stroke 2015;46(7):2032–60.
13. Connolly ES Jr, Rabinstein AA, Carhuapoma JR, et al. Guidelines for the management of aneurysmal subarachnoid hemorrhage: a guideline for healthcare professionals from the American Heart Association/American Stroke Association. Stroke 2012;43(6):1711–37.
14. Brain Trauma Foundation, American Association of Neurological Surgeons, Congress of Neurological Surgeons. Guidelines for the management of severe traumatic brain injury. Introduction. J Neurotrauma 2007;24(Suppl 1):S1–2.
15. National Collaborating Center for Acute Care. Head injury: triage, assessment, investigation and early management of head injury in infants, children and adults. London: National Collaborating Center for Acute Care; 2014.
16. Stroke Unit Trialists' Collaboration. Organised inpatient (stroke unit) care for stroke. Cochrane Database Syst Rev 2013;(9):CD000197.
17. Lang JM, Meixensberger J, Unterberg AW, et al. Neurosurgical intensive care unit–essential for good outcomes in neurosurgery? Langenbecks Arch Surg 2011;396(4):447–51.
18. Nye BR, Hyde CE, Tsivgoulis G, et al. Slim stroke scales for assessing patients with acute stroke: ease of use or loss of valuable assessment data? Am J Crit Care 2012;21(6):442–7 [quiz: 448].
19. Stone JJ, Childs S, Smith LE, et al. Hourly neurologic assessments for traumatic brain injury in the ICU. Neurol Res 2014;36(2):164–9.
20. Skoglund K, Enblad P, Hillered L, et al. The neurological wake-up test increases stress hormone levels in patients with severe traumatic brain injury. Crit Care Med 2012;40(1):216–22.
21. Teasdale G, Maas A, Lecky F, et al. The Glasgow Coma Scale at 40 years: standing the test of time. Lancet Neurol 2014;13(8):844–54.
22. Hand B, Page SJ, White S. Stroke survivors scoring zero on the NIH stroke scale score still exhibit significant motor impairment and functional limitation. Stroke Res Treat 2014;2014:462681.

Blood Pressure Management Controversies in Neurocritical Care

Molly McNett, PhD, RN, CNRN[a],*, Jay Koren, BSN, RN[b]

KEYWORDS

- Neurocritical care • Blood pressure • Monitoring • Treatment

KEY POINTS

- Blood pressure (BP) management is essential in neurocritical care settings to ensure adequate cerebral perfusion and prevent secondary brain injury. However, significant practice variations persist regarding optimal methods for monitoring and treatment of BP values among critically ill patients with neurologic injuries.
- Controversies in management include identifying optimal methods for BP monitoring and treatment. Monitoring centers on how BP is measured and recorded, whereas treatment includes use of pharmacologic agents.
- Although there is little research evidence and few recommendations to guide monitoring and treatment decisions in neurocritical care, preliminary studies support the need for ongoing research efforts. Technological advances in neurocritical care may also address aspects of controversies by providing solutions to overcome limitations of various management approaches.

INTRODUCTION

Blood pressure (BP) management is a mainstay of treatment of neurocritically ill patients. Management includes methods for monitoring BP, as well as treatment approaches to keep pressures within set parameters. Optimization of BP to ensure accordance with prescribed parameters is important for cerebral perfusion, oxygenation, and prevention of secondary brain injury. Primary injury to the brain results from hemorrhage caused by trauma, stroke, or aneurysm rupture, or ischemic events such as stroke or hypoxic episodes.[1] Secondary brain injury occurs in the

Disclosure: The authors have nothing to disclose.
[a] Nursing Research, The MetroHealth System, Nursing Business Office, 2500 MetroHealth Drive, Cleveland, OH 44109, USA; [b] Surgical Intensive Care Unit, The MetroHealth System, Nursing Business Office, 2500 MetroHealth Drive, Cleveland, OH 44109, USA
* Corresponding author.
E-mail address: mmcnett@metrohealth.org

hours and days after the initial injury and is caused by complex biochemical and physiologic responses to the initial injury, such as cellular excitotoxicity, free radical production, electrolyte shifts, inflammation, and ischemia.[1] Cerebral autoregulation in the vasculature of the brain maintains constant cerebral blood flow independently of systemic factors. However, autoregulatory mechanisms in neurocritically ill patients are often impaired by primary and secondary brain injuries. Therefore, diligent management of systemic BP becomes critical to ensure adequate cerebral perfusion.

Although there is consensus that BP management is an important element of neurocritical care, significant variations persist among practitioners and institutions with regard to how BP is monitored and treated.[2–4] Variations are caused by differences in training, fragmented research efforts, and lack of definitive practice recommendations for specific aspects of BP management among neurocritically ill patients. Variations in practice highlight the need for an evidence-based review to move toward a systematic and standardized approach to BP management. Therefore, this article is highlights management controversies for BP control in neurocritical care, and presents an evidence-based review of current practices for both monitoring and treatment.

CONTROVERSIES IN MONITORING: NONINVASIVE OR INVASIVE BLOOD PRESSURE MEASUREMENT

The initial step in identifying optimal approaches for BP management in neurocritical care is to identify the most effective approach for monitoring BP. A key controversy is whether noninvasive monitoring is comparable with invasive arterial monitoring when trending and recording BP in neurocritically ill patients. The most common noninvasive BP monitoring includes aneroid (mercury), and oscillometric (automated) BP measurement that is obtained via noninvasive cuffs.

Aneroid methods were established in the mid to late 1800s with the creation of the mercury monometer. Adaptations of the device and development of the sphygmograph throughout the 1800s resulted in a BP armband that is similar to what is still used for noninvasive manual BP monitoring.[5] In 1905, Korotkoff established the gold standard of measuring noninvasive BP with an armband, referred to as the manual auscultatory technique. The technique has 5 phases and involves inflating a cuff on the proximal arm, auscultating for phase I, which is a tapping sound and reflects systolic pressure. The diastolic pressure is determined by the disappearance of muffled sounds of phase IV. Although this technique is considered to be the gold standard for noninvasive measurements, it has limitations, such as human error when identifying auscultated sounds, cuff size error, and lack of continuous or ongoing measurements.[6]

In contrast with the manual approach for BP measurement, oscillometric BP measurement was established in 1885 with the use of sensors to detect oscillations in BP.[5] The oscillometric technique was developed before Korotkoff's auscultation method and continues to be used in current automated noninvasive BP equipment. Automated oscillometric cuffed equipment inflates to a pressure greater than systolic pressure and slowly deflates while sensors oscillate to determine resistance or pressure. The mean pressure is detected at the maximal oscillation when the artery is most compliant, and the systolic and diastolic pressures are then calculated by the equipment. Automated cuffs can be set to repeat at determined intervals but are inaccurate at intervals less than 30 seconds. As with other noninvasive techniques, there are limitations with this approach that center on human error, cuff sizing, lack of continuous readings, as well the added risk that repeated use on the same extremity can cause injury.[6]

In contrast with noninvasive BP monitoring, invasive intra-arterial monitoring provides direct measurement of BP via a catheter placed in the radial or brachial artery that is connected via a fluid column to a pressure transducer.[5] BP readings are obtained continuously and displayed on a bedside monitor. Although this approach offers additional benefits, such as an inherent line for obtaining arterial blood samples, particularly arterial blood gases, the consistent placement of a catheter within the artery poses risks such as infection, and potential damage to the arterial wall or excessive bleeding if the catheter is inadvertently removed or dislodged. In addition, skilled personnel are needed for accurate placement of the monitoring device.[5]

There are several studies that compare noninvasive BP cuff readings with those obtained by invasive arterial monitoring. Standardized guidelines for validating BP techniques are incorporated in most studies comparing BP measurement methods.[7] **Table 1** provides a summary of studies and findings. Among general critical care populations, research indicates that both manual and oscillometric BP measurements underestimate BP readings compared with invasive arterial lines.[8–11] Only 2 studies specifically compare monitoring approaches among neurocritically ill patients.[12,13] Simultaneous arterial line and oscillometric cuff pressures from 51 patients with stroke in one study indicate adequate correlations between pressures $(r = 0.85–0.88)$.[12] However, there are significant discrepancies between diastolic BP (DBP) and systolic BP (SBP) readings for each method, particularly in the presence of increased BP values. Similarly, a separate study of 301 paired measurements among postoperative neurosurgical patients compares oscillometric and arterial BPs.[13] Correlations between values are low $(r = 0.62–0.68)$, with large discrepancies between DBP, SBP, and mean arterial pressure (MAP) values. Among all populations, discrepancies are more pronounced in the presence of hypertension[8,9,12,14] and, in some instances, hypotension.[15]

Research findings suggest that invasive arterial monitoring remains a superior approach for BP monitoring, particularly in neurocritical care. However, a recent practice survey shows that up to 71% of providers continue to use noninvasive BP monitoring in the critical care setting,[4] likely because of the difficulty and skill required for placing invasive arterial lines, as well as increased risk of infection. Because noninvasive BP monitoring remains a frequently used option for practitioners despite research evidence to the contrary, newer technologies are proposed that offer continuous arterial BP monitoring without invasive catheters.

Radial artery applanation is one noninvasive approach for continuous arterial monitoring. In this technique, tonometers are placed over a superficial artery that has bony support, typically the radial artery.[16] The pressure transducer on the skin then measures arterial BP via contact pressure, also referred to as the pulse pressure method. A systematic review of research comparing noninvasive arterial monitoring with standard invasive methods included 28 studies with 919 subjects.[17] Discrepancies between recorded values averaged from 1.6 mm Hg for SBP, 5.3 mm Hg for DBP, and 3.2 mm Hg for MAP values. Ultimately the precision and accuracy of the noninvasive devices proved unacceptable in preliminary practice studies. However, 2 additional studies have since compared the two methods and reported smaller discrepancies among values.[18,19] Thus, additional revisions to the noninvasive arterial monitoring devices may yield more acceptable values in the future.

Cumulative research findings support the use of invasive arterial BP monitoring as the most accurate method for critically ill patients. Although current practice

Table 1
Summary of research comparing BP techniques

Study	Population	Methods	Findings
Penny et al[8]	N = 13 obstetric ICU patients	Repeated measures within-group comparison. Compared manual and oscillometric BP with A-line	Manual and oscillometric underestimated SBP and MAP (18–32 mm Hg); less accurate for hypertension
Araghi et al[9]	N = 54 obese ICU patients	Prospective observational study; compared manual and oscillometric BP with A-line	Manual and oscillometric underestimated A-line readings; less accurate for hypertensive patients
Muecke et al[10]	N = 18 ICU patients	Repeated measures within-group paired measurements. Compared 3 oscillometric devices with A-line	No device measured SBP accurately; MAP readings were comparable
Ribezzo et al[11]	N = 50 ICU patients	Randomized crossover trial. Compared manual and oscillometric with A-line	Manual underestimated SBP (9 mm Hg) and overestimated DBP and MAP (2–5 mm Hg); oscillometric underestimated (5–10 mm Hg) SBP; overestimated DBP
Manios et al[12]	N = 51 patients with stroke within 3 hours of onset	Repeated measures within-group comparison. Compared oscillometric with A-line	Oscillometric underestimated A-line SBP (9.7 mm Hg; P<.0001; r = 0.854–0.832). Higher discrepancies in hypertension (SBP>180 mm Hg)
Mireles et al[13]	N = 11 neurosurgical patients	Paired measurements for oscillometric and A-line evaluated using accuracy standards	Oscillometric overestimated A-line SBP 56% of the time (5 mm Hg); underestimated MAP 73% of the time (r = 0.62–0.68)

Abbreviations: A-line, arterial line; DBP, diastolic BP; ICU, intensive care unit; MAP, mean arterial pressures; SBP, systolic BP.

Data from Refs.[8–13]

guidelines do not specify the type of monitoring device that should be routinely used in all critical care settings, a recent statement from the Neurocritical Care Society recommends invasive monitoring of arterial BP in unstable patients or those at high risk for neurologic or systemic deterioration.[20]

Benefits associated with the use of invasive arterial BP monitoring, specifically accuracy of readings and accessibility for blood draws, must be weighed against the potential risks associated with insertion of the device and ongoing infection or hemorrhage risks during monitoring. Invasive approaches for BP monitoring in critical care are most appropriate in unstable patients, when vasoactive medications are being titrated, in obese patients in whom cuff size may be difficult to accurately ascertain, and when treating BP to maintain within set thresholds.[8–15,20] Specifically in neurocritical care, there are additional indications for invasive arterial BP monitoring when cerebral perfusion pressure (CPP) values are being monitored.

CONTROVERSIES IN MONITORING: ARTERIAL TRANSDUCER PLACEMENT

A second controversy in BP monitoring in neurocritical care centers on optimal placement of the transducer when invasive arterial BP monitoring is in place and being used to calculate CPP values.[21–23] Transducer placement is important in any critical care setting, because it provides the reference point from which to level the device when continuously monitoring BP. The most common location for transducer placement is the phlebostatic axis, which is located at the fourth intercostal space, midaxillary line. Leveling the arterial transducer at this location may provide the most accurate measurement of arterial BP, because it coincides with the pressures in the right atrium. However, recent surveys indicate that some critical care practitioners level the arterial transducer at the catheter insertion site, despite little evidence and few recommendations to support this practice.[21–25]

Few studies compare BP readings when the arterial transducer is placed in different reference points. One study of 29 cardiac intensive care unit (ICU) patients compares MAP readings with the arterial transducer at the midaxillary line and at the catheter site, with patients in 2 different positions (supine and semi-Fowler).[26] Correlations between readings at both sites in all positions are high ($r>0.9$), indicating little variation in readings with transducer or patient position.[26] Separate studies in animal models compare MAP in pigs placed in supine, reverse Trendelenburg, and Trendelenburg positions. The most accurate BP values were obtained with the transducer at the midaxillary line, because this coincided with pressure sensed by baroreceptor mechanisms.[27] A separate recommendation by Munis and Lozada[28] supports midaxillary transducer placement because of the state of hydrostatic indifference that occurs as long as central venous pressure and arterial transducers remain at the same level.

Specifically in neurocritical care, many practitioners level the arterial transducer at the external auditory meatus of the ear, or tragus, particularly when calculating CPP.[22–24] CPP is calculated as the mathematical difference between MAP and intracranial pressure (ICP) (MAP − ICP = CPP), and thus depends on systemic BP readings. The rationale behind leveling the arterial transducer at the tragus when calculating CPP is that measurement at this reference point provides an indication of cerebral perfusion, resulting in more accurate values when calculating CPP. Surveys of nurses, advanced practice providers, and physicians practicing in neurointensive care units indicate that 25% to 41% level the arterial transducer at the tragus,[22–25] whereas 62% to 74% level the transducer at the midaxillary line[22–24] when calculating CPP.

There is little evidence to guide recommendations regarding placement of the arterial transducer when recording MAP values that are then used to calculate CPP. A statement from 1959 indicates that CPP should be measured using MAP obtained at the foramen of Monro (tragus), rather than at the level of the heart.[29] However, there is no evidence to substantiate this claim, and no evidence directing location of measurement for optimal CPP therapy. Parameters become particularly important if a physiologic transducer is lower than the true reference point. In this scenario, there is an increase in hydrostatic pressure, and a higher value is reported. In contrast, if a transducer is higher than the true reference point, hydrostatic pressure is decreased, resulting in a lower value. As a result, false high values for MAP result in false high values for CPP, placing the patient at risk for cerebral hypoperfusion and ischemia. For example, if a patient head of bed is at 50°, measuring MAP at the midaxillary region could result in a calculated CPP up to 15 mm Hg higher than CPP values obtained when MAP is measured at the tragus.[30,31] Therefore, there may be a CPP reading of 60 mm Hg at the midaxillary level when the true CPP is 45 mm Hg, causing severe cerebral ischemia because of incorrect reporting and treating of a CPP calculated at 60 mm Hg.

Evidence is needed to guide practice recommendations for optimal arterial BP transducer location when calculating CPP in neurocritically ill patients. Current research is intended to identify specific variations in readings based on transducer location in neurocritical care, and the implications of these readings for CPP management (McNett MM, Olson DW, unpublished data, 2015). An investigation of various approaches on patient outcomes will provide the needed evidence to move toward best practice recommendations regarding optimal location for BP monitoring in the neurocritical care setting.

Additional research efforts in neurocritical care are evaluating technological advances to determine alternate methods of measuring CPP and autoregulatory mechanisms.[32–35] Use of a pressure reactivity index (PRx) is an alternate approach to traditional CPP monitoring and provides an indication of cerebral autoregulatory capacity. PRx values are calculated as a correlation coefficient between average ICP values and mean arterial BPs over 5-second periods.[34] PRx values can be used to determine optimal CPP values for each patient, rather than relying on set thresholds across populations.[34,35] Integration of this technology may have important implications for BP monitoring, because BP thresholds may not play as crucial a role because of newer technologies that target optimal CPP metrics. Research evaluating the effectiveness of this technology on specific neurocritical care populations is warranted, along with studies to evaluate feasibility and integration into routine clinical care.

CONTROVERSIES IN BLOOD PRESSURE MANAGEMENT: TREATMENT

In addition to BP monitoring controversies, there are also variations in how to effectively manage BP. Identification of optimal pharmacologic agents for BP control remains elusive, along with consensus on methods for delivery of these agents. Among general critical care patients, initial medications to manage severe hypertension include labetalol, nicardipine, hydralazine, and sodium nitroprusside.[36] Specifically among neurocritically patients with spontaneous intracerebral hemorrhage, nicardipine and labetalol are used most often.[37] Both labetalol and nicardipine remain preferred agents for BP control among patients with ischemic stroke.[38] However, there remain few data on the efficacy of these different agents and the impact of agents on BP variability. A recent systematic review compared nicardipine and labetalol by examining 10 studies.[39] Efficacy of agents on acute hypertension was examined across diagnosis types and treatment settings. Conclusions indicate that these agents have comparable safety and efficacy; however, nicardipine seems to show more predictable and consistent BP control.

Table 2 provides a summary of additional research comparing the two pharmacologic agents specifically within neurocritical care populations. Consensus based on cumulative findings from these studies indicates that both nicardipine and labetalol are effective agents for BP control in neurocritical care[40–44]; however, nicardipine may elicit a faster BP response and less BP variability when used in this patient population.[43–47] There remains a need for prospective randomized trials to effectively evaluate each agent before definitive practice recommendations can be made.

Within pharmacologic administration of labetalol and nicardipine, there is also controversy regarding route of delivery. Studies listed in **Table 2** specifically examine medications administered intermittently via intravenous bolus or by continuous infusion. Cumulative findings from studies indicate that neither route is consistently superior for administration of these pharmacologic agents in neurocritical care.[40–47] Either route may elicit similar results for BP control. Again, well-designed randomized trials comparing pharmacologic agents that include various routes of administration are needed to better define practice guidelines for BP control in neurocritical care populations.

RECOMMENDATIONS, FUTURE RESEARCH, AND TECHNOLOGICAL ADVANCES

There remains a lack of evidence-based recommendations regarding specific approaches for BP monitoring in neurocritical care. Current recommendations all indicate that continuous BP monitoring is a key component of care for critically ill patients with neurologic injury.[20,48,49] Recommendations from the Neurocritical Care Society are the only ones to date that designate a specific method of monitoring BP. The recommendation is for use of invasive arterial monitoring, but only for unstable patients or those at risk for acute deterioration.[20] The choice of BP monitoring approach in neurocritical care remains primarily rooted in provider preferences and patient condition. However, there is evidence that invasive arterial monitoring remains the gold standard and most accurate method for monitoring BP in neurocritically ill patients, particularly in the presence of hypertension.

When invasive arterial monitoring is used for BP measurement, additional evidence is needed to support recommendations regarding optimal placement of the transducer when calculating CPP in neurocritically ill patients. Current research is evaluating these differences, and technological advances in neuromonitoring may influence future practices.

Neuromonitoring continues to grow substantially.[32] Devices for noninvasive arterial BP measurement may yield alternate approaches for BP monitoring that offer benefits of traditional invasive monitoring, but without the risks associated with use of indwelling catheters.[6] In addition, proposed technologies for measurement of cerebrovascular reactivity, perfusion, and oxygenation[32,35] may offer additional parameters that supersede traditional calculations of CPP that are based on ICP and BP values.[50] Research is needed to evaluate these new technologies not only for comparison with established gold standards but also for effects on patient outcomes and the feasibility of routine use in clinical care.

Table 2
Summary of research comparing labetalol and nicardipine

Study	Population	Methods	Findings
Kross et al[40]	N = 42 craniotomy patients for tumor removal	RCT; compared IV bolus nicardipine to bolus labetalol postoperatively with enalaprilat for emergence hypertension	Labetalol more effective at BP reduction; (99%), compared with nicardipine (90%)
Powers et al[41]	N = 14 with nontraumatic intracerebral hemorrhage	RCT; compared nicardipine bolus/infusion to labetalol bolus	Both effective for BP targets; no difference in cerebral blood flow. Nicardipine required less fentanyl
Martin-Schild et al[42]	N = 50 acute ischemic stroke	Retrospective; compared labetalol bolus, labetalol/nicardipine infusion, nicardipine infusion	Both agents effective for BP targets. Patients given nicardipine had shorter lengths of stay
Liu-DeRyke et al[43]	N = 90 patients with stroke	Retrospective; compared nicardipine infusion with labetalol boluses	Nicardipine group had less BP variability, fewer dosage adjustments, fewer additional antihypertensive agents. For intracerebral hemorrhage: 33% of nicardipine group reached target BP in 60 minutes, compared with 6% of labetalol group
Malesker & Killeman[45]	N = 382 ICU patients	Retrospective; compared continuous infusion nicardipine with continuous/intermittent labetalol	One-third of subjects had neurologic diagnosis. Nicardipine group had better BP target (83% vs 67%, $P = .04$), fewer patients needing alternate antihypertensives (31% vs 17%; $P = .02$), and fewer adverse events (61% vs 48%, $P = .04$)
Woloszyn et al[46]	N = 103 aneurysmal subarachnoid hemorrhage	Retrospective; compared labetalol prn with continuous nicardipine	Nicardipine had longer time within goal MAP and more rapid response to therapy
Ortega-Gutierrez et al[44]	N = 81 subarachnoid hemorrhage; intracerebral hemorrhage	Retrospective; compared continuous nicardipine, labetalol, and combination nicardipine/labetalol	No difference in median BP variability, hypotension, bradycardia; mean time to goal was faster for nicardipine group (32 vs 53 min, $P = .003$)
Liu-DeRyke et al[47]	N = 54 patients with stroke in emergency department	Prospective pseudorandomized study. Compared labetalol bolus with nicardipine infusion	BP goal higher for nicardipine (100% vs 89%). 89% of nicardipine at goal in 60 min vs 25% in labetalol group; less antihypertensive agent given to nicardipine group; no difference in clinical outcomes

Abbreviations: IV, intravenous; prn, as needed; RCT, randomized controlled trial.
Data from Refs.[40–47]

SUMMARY

Although controversies for BP management continue in neurocritical care, evidence is emerging to guide recommendations for clinicians in both monitoring and treatment. Technological advances that address controversies in monitoring need to be evaluated for both effectiveness and clinical utility. Research is needed to fully delineate optimal approaches for BP management and provide a solid evidence base to guide future recommendations.

REFERENCES

1. American Association of Neuroscience Nurses. Core curriculum for neuroscience nursing. Philadelphia: Lippincott; 2010.
2. Olson D, Lewis L, Bader M, et al. Significant practice pattern variations associated with intracranial pressure monitoring. J Neurosci Nurs 2013;45(4):186–93.
3. Olson DM, Batjer HH, Abdulkadir K, et al. Measuring and monitoring ICP in neurocritical care: results from a national practice survey. Neurocrit Care 2014;20(1): 15–20.
4. Chatterjee A, DePriest K, Blair R, et al. Results of a survey of blood pressure monitoring by intensivists in critically ill patients: a preliminary study. Crit Care Med 2010;38:2335–8.
5. O'Brien E, Fitzgerald D. The history of blood pressure measurement. J Hum Hypertens 1994;8(2):73–84.
6. Smulyan H, Safar M. Blood pressure management: retrospective and prospective views. Am J Hypertens 2011;24(6):628–34.
7. Obrien E, Picker T, Asmar R, et al. Working group on blood pressure monitoring of the European Society of Hypertension international protocol for validation of blood pressure measuring devices in adults. Blood Press Monit 2002;7:3–17.
8. Penny JA, Shennan AH, Halligan AW, et al. The relative accuracy of sequential same-arm and simultaneous opposite-arm measurements for the intra-arterial validation of blood pressure monitors. Blood Press Monit 1999;4:91–5.
9. Araghi A, Bander J, Guzman JA. Arterial blood pressure monitoring in overweight critically ill patients: invasive or noninvasive? Crit Care 2006;10(2):R64.
10. Muecke S, Bersten A, Plummer J. The mean machine: accurate non-invasive blood pressure measurement in the critically ill patient. J Clin Monit Comput 2009;23:283–97.
11. Ribezzo S, Spina E, Di Bartolomeo S, et al. Noninvasive techniques for blood pressure measurement are not a reliable alternative to direct measurement: a randomized crossover trial in the ICU. ScientificWorldJournal 2014;2014:353628, 1–8.
12. Manios E, Vemmos K, Tsivgoulis G, et al. Comparison of noninvasive oscillometric and intra-arterial blood pressure measurements in hyperacute stroke. Blood Press Monit 2007;12:149–56.
13. Mireles SA, Jaffe RA, Drover DR, et al. A poor correlation exists between oscillometric and radial arterial blood pressure as measured by the Philips MP90 monitor. J Clin Monit Comput 2009;23:169–74.
14. Braam RL, Thien T. Is the accuracy of blood pressure measuring devices underestimated at increasing blood pressure levels? Blood Press Monit 2005;10:283–9.
15. Davis JW, Davis IC, Bennink LD, et al. Are automated blood pressure measurements accurate in trauma patients? J Trauma 2003;55:860–3.
16. Chung E, Chen G, Alexander B, et al. Non-invasive continuous blood pressure monitoring: a review of current applications. Front Med 2013;7(1):91–101.

17. Kim SH, Lilot M, Sidhu KS, et al. Accuracy and precision of continuous noninvasive arterial pressure monitoring compared with invasive arterial pressure. Anesthesiology 2014;120:1080–97.
18. Peterson NH, Ortega-Gutierrez S, Reccius A, et al. Comparison of non-invasive and invasive arterial blood pressure measurement for assessment of dynamic cerebral autoregulation. Neurocrit Care 2014;20(1):60–8.
19. Meidert AS, Lilot M, Sidhu KS, et al. Radial artery applanation tonometry for continuous non-invasive arterial pressure monitoring in intensive care unit patients: comparison with invasively assessed radial arterial pressure. Br J Anaesth 2014;112(3):521–8.
20. Taccone F, Citerio G. Advanced monitoring of systemic hemodynamics in critically ill patients with acute brain injury. Neurocrit Care 2014;21:S38–63.
21. Nates JL, Niggemeyer LE, Anderson MB, et al. Cerebral perfusion pressure monitoring alert! Crit Care Med 1997;25(5):895–6.
22. Kosty JA, Leroux PD, Levine J, et al. Brief report: a comparison of clinical and research practices in measuring cerebral perfusion pressure: a literature review and practitioner survey. Anesth Analg 2013;117(3):694–8.
23. Rao V, Klepstad P, Losvik O, et al. Confusion with cerebral perfusion pressure in a literature review of current guidelines and survey of clinical practice. Scand J Trauma Resusc Emerg Med 2013;21:78–82.
24. Jones, HA. Cerebral perfusion pressure and arterial transducer level. BACCN conference presentation. York, UK, September 15, 2008.
25. Ingram M, Lightfoot R, Eynon A. Survey of cerebral perfusion pressure measurement: location of the arterial transducer in the patient managed at 30 degrees elevation. Crit Care 2006;(Suppl 1):450.
26. Kirchoff K, Rebenson-Piano M, Patel M. Mean arterial pressure readings: variations with positions and transducer level. Nurs Res 1984;33(6):343–5.
27. McCann U, Schiller HJ, Carney DE, et al. Invasive arterial BP monitoring in trauma and critical care: effect of variable transducer level, catheter access, and patient position. Chest 2001;120(4):1322–6.
28. Munis J, Lozada LJ. Giraffes, siphons and starling resistors: cerebral perfusion pressure revisited. J Neurosurg Anesthesiol 2000;12:290–6.
29. Lassen NA. Cerebral blood flow and oxygen consumption in man. Physiol Rev 1959;39(2):183–238.
30. Pohl A, Cullen DJ. Cerebral ischemia during shoulder surgery in the upright position: a case series. J Clin Anesth 2005;17(6):463–9.
31. Rosner MJ, Coley IB. Cerebral perfusion pressure, intracranial pressure, and head elevation. J Neurosurg 1986;65(5):636–41.
32. Mahdavi Z, Pierre-Louis N, Ho TT, et al. Advances in cerebral monitoring for the patient with traumatic brain injury. Crit Care Nurs Clin North Am 2015;27: 213–23.
33. Lang E, Kasprowicz M, Smielewshi P, et al. Changes in cerebral partial oxygen pressure and cerebrovascular reactivity during intracranial pressure plateau waves. Neurocrit Care 2015;23:85–91.
34. Depreitere B, Guiza F, Van den Berghe G, et al. Pressure autoregulation monitoring and cerebral perfusion pressure target recommendation in patients with severe traumatic brain injury based on minute-by-minute monitoring data. J Neurosurg 2014;120(6):1451–7.
35. Lang EW, Kasprowicz M, Smielewski P, et al. Short pressure reactivity index versus long pressure reactivity index in the management of traumatic brain injury. J Neurosurg 2015;122(3):588–94.

36. Mayer SA, Kurtz P, Wyman A, et al. Clinical practices, complications, and mortality in neurological patients with acute severe hypertension: the studying the treatment of acute hypertension registry. Crit Care Med 2011;39(10):2330–6.
37. Anderson CS, Heeley E, Huang Y, et al. Rapid blood-pressure lowering in patients with acute intracerebral hemorrhage. N Engl J Med 2013;368(25):2355–65.
38. American Heart Association, American Stroke Association. Guidelines for the early management of patients with acute ischemic stroke. Stroke 2013;44: 870–947.
39. Peacock WF, Hilleman DE, Levey PD, et al. A systematic review of nicardipine vs. labetalol for the management of hypertensive crises. Am J Emerg Med 2012;30: 981–93.
40. Kross RA, Ferri E, Leung D, et al. A comparative study between a calcium channel blocker (nicardipine) and a combined alpha/beta blocker (labetalol) for the control of emergence hypertension during craniotomy for tumor surgery. Anesth Analg 2000;91:904–9.
41. Powers WJ, Zazulia AR, Videen TO, et al. Autoregulation of cerebral blood flow surrounding acute intracerebral hemorrhage. Neurology 2001;57:18–24.
42. Martin-Schild S, Hallevi H, Allbright KC, et al. Aggressive blood pressure-lowering treatment before tissue plasminogen activator therapy in acute ischemic stroke. Arch Neurol 2008;65:1174–8.
43. Liu-DeRyke X, Coplin JJ, Parker D, et al. A comparison of nicardipine and labetalol for acute hypertension management following stroke. Neurocrit Care 2008;9(2): 167–76.
44. Ortega-Gutierrez S, Thomas J, Reccius A, et al. Effectiveness and safety of nicardipine and labetalol infusion for blood pressure management in patients with intracerebral and subarachnoid hemorrhage. Neurocrit Care 2013;18(1):13–9.
45. Malesker MA, Killeman DE. Intravenous labetalol compared with intravenous nicardipine in the management of hypertension in critically ill patients. J Crit Care 2012;27:528e1–528e14.
46. Woloszyn AV, McAllen KJ, Figueroa BE, et al. Retrospective evaluation of nicardipine versus labetalol for blood pressure control in aneurysmal subarachnoid hemorrhage. Neurocrit Care 2012;16(3):376–80.
47. Liu-DeRyke X, Levy PD, Parker D, et al. A prospective evaluation of labetalol versus nicardipine for blood pressure management of patients with acute stroke. Neurocrit Care 2013;19:41–7.
48. Bratton SL, Chestnut RM, Ghajar J, et al. Guidelines for the management of severe traumatic brain injury. Blood pressure and oxygenation. J Neurotrauma 2007; 24(Suppl 1):S59–64.
49. Ciccone A, Celani M, Chiaramonte R, et al. Continuous versus intermittent physiological monitoring for acute stroke. Cochrane Database Syst Rev 2013;(5):CD008444.
50. Kirkman MA, Smith M. Intracranial pressure monitoring, cerebral perfusion pressure estimation, and ICP/CPP-guided therapy: a standard of care or optional extra after traumatic brain injury? Br J Anaesth 2014;112(1):35–46.

Delirium in the Neuro Intensive Care Unit

Joseph B. Haymore, MS, ACNP-BC[a,b,*], Nikhil Patel, MD, MBA[c]

KEYWORDS

- Delirium • Inattention • Altered level of consciousness • Validated tools
- Assessment

KEY POINTS

- Delirium in the neuro intensive care unit (ICU) affects as many as 10% to 48% of patients.
- There are few studies looking specifically at the neuro ICU patient population and delirium; thus, nurses rely on general ICU data to make evidence-based decisions.
- Delirium cannot be addressed without also monitoring pain, sedation, and agitation using validated tools.
- The Confusion Assessment Method for the ICU and the Intensive Care Delirium Screening Checklist are the validated delirium assessment tools recommended by national guidelines.

Delirium is a common, serious, and life-threatening complication in the intensive care unit (ICU). Nurses should assess their patients for delirium risk factors, appropriately assess for and manage pain and sedation or agitation, and monitor for the emergence of delirium with all patients. To properly assess and monitor for this critical patient safety condition, nurses must use appropriate, validated assessment tools and not rely solely on clinical observations and judgment.

Delirium is in many ways similar to acute kidney injury (AKI). The modern ICU nurse and clinical team is aware that their patients are at high risk of AKI, with 20% to 50% of the patients having some degree of AKI during their time in the ICU.[1] By being aware of which patients are at risk for AKI, avoiding interventions that put the patient at increased risk, regularly monitoring renal function, and intervening early when signs of renal end-organ dysfunction are noticed, the clinical team will improve that patient's likelihood of either not developing AKI or having a limited course with full recovery. Delirium is also common, affecting 20% to greater than 80% of ICU patients. Delirium is an acute brain injury, a manifestation of end-organ dysfunction or damage owing to a combination of the patient's own

Disclosures: None.
[a] Neurocritical Care Unit, University of Maryland Medical Center, 22 South Greene Street, Baltimore, MD, USA; [b] University of Maryland School of Nursing, 655 West Lombard Street, Baltimore, MD 21201, USA; [c] Department of Neurology, University of Maryland School of Medicine, 620 West Lexington Street, Baltimore, MD 21201, USA
* Corresponding author.
E-mail address: jhaymore@umm.edu

Crit Care Nurs Clin N Am 28 (2016) 21–35
http://dx.doi.org/10.1016/j.cnc.2015.11.001
0899-5885/16/$ – see front matter © 2016 Elsevier Inc. All rights reserved.
ccnursing.theclinics.com

risk factors and the effects of acute illness. Many patients with delirium recover and have few if any long-term complications. However, some will experience long-term, often permanent cognitive impairment, namely, chronic brain failure. The ICU nurse should view the acutely ill patient as being at risk for any end-organ dysfunction (eg, lung, heart, skin) and routinely monitor the patient based on the best available evidence.

Delirium in the neuro ICU setting is an especially challenging condition. Most patients admitted to a neuro ICU have some degree of brain dysfunction due to an illness, condition, or trauma. Because delirium is an acute brain injury, it can be difficult to determine whether the patient's behavior is because of her hemorrhage, stroke, meningitis, or other factor, or that she is developing an additional brain dysfunction in the form of delirium. It is this difficulty with teasing out delirium from the primary brain dysfunction that most of the research into delirium in the ICU has been conducted in the medical, surgical, and cardiothoracic ICU settings. Therefore, the majority of the information in this article is pertinent to all ICUs. The data specific to the neuro ICU setting are discussed when available. This article discusses what delirium is and who is at risk, and reviews the process of monitoring patients in the ICU for delirium. The appropriate assessment tools for each step of the monitoring process are described.

WHAT IS DELIRIUM?

Delirium is a behavioral syndrome that includes an altered level of consciousness (LOC), difficulty maintaining attention, and a change in cognition or perception. The onset is acute (hours to days) and has a fluctuating course that might include periods of lucid, normal mental functioning. The behavior must be owing to a medical condition, use of a medication or other substance (ie, alcohol or recreational drugs), or withdrawal from a medication or substance, but not owing to a primary psychiatric condition (**Table 1**).[2]

Delirium Motor Subtypes

Patients with delirium may be consistently hyperactive or agitated (<2%), hypoactive or withdrawn (44%–68%), or have a mixture of hyperactivity and hypoactivity over the

Table 1		
Motor subtype classification–characteristic behaviors		
Hyperactive	**Hypoactive[a]**	**Mixed**
Increased activity levels	Decreased amount of activity	At least 1 behavior noted from each of the hyperactive and hypoactive characteristics
Increased speed of actions	Decreased speed of actions	
Loss of control of activity	Reduced awareness of surroundings	
Restlessness		
Wandering	Decreased amount of speech	
Increased speed of speech	Decreased speed of speech	
Hyperalertness	Decreased volume of speech	
Fear	Apathy/listlessness	
Uncooperativeness	Reduced alertness/withdrawal	
Combativeness		

[a] At least 1 of either decreased amount of motor activity or speed of actions is present.

Adapted from Meagher D, Moran M, Raju B, et al. A new data-based motor subtype schema for delirium. J Neuropsychiatry Clin Neurosci 2008; 20(2):190; with permission.

course of a day (31%-55%).[3–5] Hyperactive delirium is usually detected earlier, precipitating factors are addressed more quickly, and the duration is shorter. Hypoactive delirium is more difficult to detect during usual clinical assessments. The patient who is quiet and withdrawn may not receive as much attention from busy clinicians and therefore have a longer duration of delirium. Robinson and colleagues[5] reported that patients aged 65 and older had a much higher rate of hypoactive delirium than those who were younger (41% vs 22%; $P<.001$) and the older group did not have any instances of pure hyperactive delirium. Mixed delirium is simply episodes of both hyperdelirium and hypodelirium during the course of a 24-hour period (see **Table 1**).

INCIDENCE AND CONSEQUENCES

Delirium is common. As many as 20% to 50% of the patients in an ICU without mechanical ventilation will have at least 1 episode of delirium during their stay. If a patient is receiving mechanical ventilation, the rate is as high as 80%.[6] In the neurocritical care setting, the occurrence of delirium is also quite common, with rates of 19% to 70% reported.[7,8]

Delirium is associated with significantly increased morbidity and mortality. Critically ill patients with delirium are almost 3 times more likely to die in the hospital. They also require more days of mechanical ventilation and have a longer duration of stay in the ICU and in hospital duration of stay.[9] Patients in the ICU who develop delirium and have delayed treatment (>24 hours after symptom onset) are 25% more likely to die, 20% more likely to develop a nosocomial infection, and 30% more likely to develop pneumonia while in the ICU.[10]

The long-term outcomes are also worse for patients with delirium. Of those patients with delirium who are discharged from the hospital, as many as 25% will die within the first 6 months. In addition, these patients are at significant risk of long-term cognitive impairment.[9] Anderson and colleagues[11] noted that elderly patients who have delirium in the hospital and are discharged to a postacute care facility, more than one-half (57%) had delirium on admission to the postacute care facility and continued to have delirium after 1 month. These patients with delirium in the postacute care setting had higher rates of pneumonia, urinary tract infections, dehydration, pressure ulcers, and falls. Because delirium is common in the ICU, and the consequences of developing delirium are significant, every ICU clinician should be aware of it, detect and treat it early, and therefore reduce the suffering of the patients and their families.

What about the psychological effects of delirium on patients and nurses (**Table 2**)? Bélanger and Ducharme[12] reviewed the limited research into this very important topic. They found that patients who survived delirium had feelings of not being able to comprehend events as they happened and a great feeling of discomfort with the experience. Patients felt that they needed to keep their distance from the staff and to do anything that they thought was self-protective (withdraw or fight back). Patients were comforted when they felt that the nurses understood them, even if the patients did not know who they were dealing with, or even why they were there.

Bélanger and Ducharme[12] also described the research on the psychological effects that nurses experienced when caring for patients with delirium. The nurses described incomprehension about their patients' behavior, especially when their patient fluctuated between delirium and lucidity. The nurses experienced distress when trying to balance the patient's need for increased time to participate in care and the freedom to expresses their needs, even if not rational, against the safety of the patients and harmony on the nursing unit. The authors demonstrated that delirium has a very confusing, frightening, and distressing psychological effect on patients and nurses.

Table 2 Patient and nurse emotional responses to delirium	
Patient	**Nurse**
Themes	
Fluctuating between confusion and comprehension	Loss of trust in the patient
Having no control over their lives	Empathy for the distress of the patient and family
Feeling that their lives, families, and values were under assault; feeling of being held captive in a dark place	Frustration with the patient's waxing and waning ability to understand and remember
In a world of distorted perceptions, hallucinations, and a never-ending nightmare	Unsure about remaining flexible or increasing control with the patient
Adjectives	
Anxious	Ambivalent
Fearful	Frustrated
Frustrated	Angry
Lost	Distrustful
Paranoid	Guilty

Data from Maldonado JR. Neuropathogenesis of delirium: review of current etiologic theories and common pathways. Am J Geriatr Psychiatry 2013;21(12):1190–222.

PATHOPHYSIOLOGY

The pathophysiology of delirium is typically multifactorial and usually occurs in patients who are predisposed to developing delirium. There is no clear single etiology of delirium, but instead a collection of mechanisms that leads to delirium. The main proposed mechanisms include[13] the neuroinflammation hypothesis, oxidative stress hypothesis, neurotransmitter hypothesis, neuroendocrine hypothesis, and neuronal aging hypothesis.

Neuroinflammation Hypothesis

Systemic inflammation (eg, infection/sepsis, surgery, trauma) leads to the release of brain proinflammatory cytokines. The activation of these brain inflammatory substances leads to brain cellular dysfunction.

Oxidative Stress Hypothesis

Hypoperfusion of tissues leads to a buildup of oxygen free radicals. If these toxic free radicals are not cleared adequately, the tissue will be further damaged. The resulting tissue damage cascade leads to an inflammatory response, first locally and ultimately systemically. Eventually the oxidative stress response will trigger the proinflammatory response.

Neurotransmitter Hypothesis

This mechanism is most often implicated in delirium owing to medication and/or recreational substance use or withdrawal. Any imbalance in the excitatory and inhibitory substances in the brain can lead to delirium through complex and interrelated interactions with specific neurotransmitters.

Neuroendocrine Hypothesis

Acute stress leads to increased levels of glucocorticoids (including cortisol), which reduces the survivability of neurons. Acute stress stimulates the hypothalamus to in turn stimulate the pituitary gland to produce adrenocorticotropic hormone. The adrenocorticotropic hormone stimulates the adrenal gland to produce glucocorticoids. These glucocorticoids assist the body and brain in coping with acute stressors. However, when present in high concentrations for a prolonged period the glucocorticoids will result in neuronal dysfunction.

Neuronal Aging Hypothesis

As people age, they experience a decline in their physiologic reserve in all systems. This decreased reserve makes patients more vulnerable to neuronal dysfunction during critical illness. This mechanism is believed to be a reason why advancing age is an independent risk factor for developing delirium.

DELIRIUM ASSESSMENT

There are multiple factors that are essential to maximize the nurse's ability to monitor patients for delirium and the resolution of delirium. Delirium monitoring is most effectively accomplished when it is viewed as a process (**Fig. 1**). The etiology of delirium is multifactorial and owing to a complex interplay between the state of the patient's health before admission to the ICU, the severity of the acute illness, and the added stressors that are found in the ICU environment.

An understanding of the patient's unique risk factors for delirium will allow the nurse to identify those patients at greatest risk, leading to heightened sensitivity to changes in the patient's behavior. The next essential step in delirium monitoring is a careful pain assessment. Inadequately treated pain not only results in patient suffering, but it also increases the risk for delirium. Once pain is assessed and treated, the clinician must assess for agitation and institute appropriate sedation strategies if indicated. Inadequate or inappropriate sedation management leads to increased patient suffering and increased risk for delirium. Lastly, patients should be routinely screened for delirium.

Step 1: Risk Factor Assessment

There are many risk factors associated with delirium. They can be broadly divided into predisposing factors and precipitating factors. Predisposing factors are the individual patient characteristics that make him vulnerable to developing delirium, namely, genetics, chronic disease, mental health history, and others. Precipitating factors are

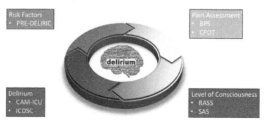

Fig. 1. Delirium assessment process. BPS, Behavioral Pain Scale; CAM-ICU, Confusion Assessment Method for the Intensive Care Unit; CPOT, Critical-care Pain Observation Tool; ICDSC, Intensive Care Delirium Screening Checklist; PRE-DELIRIC, PREdiction of DELIRium in ICu patients; RASS, Richmond Agitation-Sedation Scale; SAS, Riker Sedation-Agitation Scale. (© Can Stock Photo Inc. /paradoxfx. Used with permission.)

the events or conditions that trigger the vulnerable patient's development of delirium (**Box 1**).

Van den Boogaard and colleagues[14,15] developed a delirium prediction tool called PREdiction of DELIRium in ICu patients (PRE-DELIRIC) that accurately predicts

---

Box 1
Risk factors for delirium

Predisposing (vulnerability) factors

- Patient characteristics
  - Age
  - Dementia
  - Depression
  - Neurologic impairment
  - Functionally dependent
  - Visual impairment
  - Hearing impairment
  - Alcohol abuse
  - Tobacco use
  - Use of psychoactive medications
  - Polypharmacy
  - Chronic disease
    - Hypertension, malnutrition, dehydration, etc
  - Immobility

Precipitating (trigger) factors

- Acute illness
- Increased illness severity
- Hypoxia
- Hypotension
- Hyperglycemia or hypoglycemia
- Uremia
- Metabolic acidosis
- Immobility
- Coma
- Extended length of stay (>5 days)
- Indwelling urinary catheters
- Admission through the emergency department
- Admission through transfer from another facility or unit
- Trauma
- Invasive procedures
- Pain
- Surgery
- Isolation
- Poor quality sunlight
- Physical restraints

Data from Refs.[14,22–24]

delirium 77% to 87% of the time. The PRE-DELIRIC uses 10 risk factors (age, Acute Physiology And Chronic Health Evaluation [APACHE]-II score, admission group, coma, infection, metabolic acidosis, use of sedatives and morphine, urea concentration, and urgent admission) to predict the likelihood of developing delirium. All of the data needed for the PRE-DELIRIC are available within 24-hours of admission in a typical ICU. This tool has been studied rigorously and validated across multiple ICU settings (medical, surgical, trauma, and neuro) and in multiple countries in Australia and multiple countries in Europe. However, there is an important caveat for using the PRE-DELIRIC in the neuro ICU setting. Of the patients studied in the development and validation of this tool, only 16% (n = 784/4880) were in a neurocritical care setting. Further research is needed before this tool can be widely used in the neuro ICU.

Steps 2: Pain Assessment

Pain is very common in the ICU, with as many as 50% of the patients experiencing pain at rest and up to 80% during routine care.[16] Poorly controlled pain (undertreated or overtreated) can both trigger the emergence of delirium and potentially interfere with monitoring, leading to a delay in detection and intervention.

The American Association of Critical-Care Nurses and the Society of Critical Care Medicine have published guidelines calling for routine monitoring of pain, using patient self-reporting of pain when possible.[17,18] Both organizations recommend using a validated behavioral pain scale to assess when a patient is unable to effectively self-report. The tools that they recommend are the Behavioral Pain Scale and the Critical-Care Pain Observation Tool (**Tables 3** and **4** respectively). These tools are a structured method of observing the patient at rest and also assessing her response to stimulation, and should be used with all routine assessments and when there is a suspicion of pain (eg, changes in activity, change in vital signs).

Step 3: Level of Consciousness—Sedation–Agitation Assessment

The next important step is to assess the patient's LOC. Consciousness has 2 major components, arousal and content. If a patient does not have an adequate level of arousal, then consciousness cannot emerge. This level of arousal is described along a continuum

Table 3 Behavioral Pain Scale (BPS)		
Assess	**Description**	**Score**
Facial expression	Relaxed	1
	Partially tense	2
	Totally tense	3
	Grimace	4
Movements of upper limbs	Relaxed	1
	Partially flexed	2
	Totally flexed	3
	Totally contracted	4
Mechanical ventilation	Tolerating movements	1
	Coughing, but tolerating during most of the time	2
	Fighting the ventilator	3
	Impossible to control the ventilator	4
Total range (higher number = more pain)		3–12

From Payen J, Bru O, Bosson J, et al. Assessing pain in critically ill sedated patients by using a behavioral pain scale. Crit Care Med 2001;29(12):2258–63; with permission.

Table 4
Critical Care Pain Observation Tool (CPOT)

Assess	Description	Label	Score
Facial expression	No muscular tension observed	Relaxed, neutral	0
	Presence of frowning, brow lowering, orbit tightening, and levator contraction	Tense	1
	All of the above facial movements plus eyelid tightly closed	Grimacing	2
Body movements	Does not move at all (does not necessarily mean absence of pain)	Absence of movements	0
	Slow, cautious movements, touching or rubbing the pain site, seeking attention through movements	Protection	1
	Pulling tube, attempting to sit up, moving limbs/not following commands, striking at staff, trying to climb out of bed	Restlessness	2
Muscle tension	No resistance to passive movements	Relaxed	0
Evaluate with passive flexion and extension of upper extremities	Resistance to passive movements	Tense, rigid	1
	Strong resistance to passive movements, inability to complete them	Very tense or rigid	2
Compliance with the ventilator (intubated patients)	Alarms not activated, easy ventilation	Tolerating ventilator	0
	Alarms stop spontaneously	Coughing but tolerating	1
	Asynchrony: blocking ventilation, alarms frequently, activated	Fighting ventilator	2
or			
Vocalization (nonintubated patients)	Talking in normal tone or no sound	Talking in normal tone or no sound	0
	Sighing, moaning	Sighing, moaning	1
	Crying out, sobbing	Crying out, sobbing	2
Total range (higher number = more pain)			3–12

From Gélinas C, Fillion L, Puntillo K. Item selection and content validity of the Critical-Care Pain Observation Tool for non-verbal adults. J Adv Nurs 2008;65(1):203–16; with permission.

from coma, to sedated, to awake and alert, to agitated, to combative and violent. The nurse needs to be aware of where her patient is along this continuum for multiple reasons. If her patient needs sedation, she must make sure that the patient is appropriately sedated. Maintaining a patient with the lightest level of sedation needed is clearly associated with earlier liberation from mechanical ventilation, fewer nosocomial infections, and a reduction in post ICU psychological and cognitive impairment.[18] The use of validated sedation–agitation tools along with daily interruptions of sedation has been shown to reduce the amount and duration of use of sedative medication across multiple settings.

The other important reason to appropriately monitor LOC is that an altered LOC is a defining characteristic of delirium. If a patient has an unexplained fluctuation in LOC, he may be developing delirium. The American Association of Critical-Care Nurses and Society of Critical Care Medicine recommend using the Richmond Agitation–Sedation Scale (RASS) and the Riker Sedation–Agitation Scale (SAS; **Tables 5** and **6** respectively).

Table 5 Richmond Agitation–Sedation Scale (RASS)				
Score	Classification	Descriptor	Motor Subtype	LOC
4	Combative	Overtly combative or violent; immediate danger to staff	Hyperactive	Altered
3	Very agitated	Pulls on or removes tube(s) or catheter(s) or has aggressive behavior toward staff		
2	Agitated	Frequent nonpurposeful movement or patient–ventilator dyssynchrony		
1	Restless	Anxious or apprehensive but movements not aggressive or vigorous		
0	Alert and calm	—	—	Not altered
−1	Drowsy	Not fully alert, but has sustained (>10 s) awakening, with eye contact, to voice	Hypoactive	Altered
−2	Light sedation	Briefly (<10 s) awakens with eye contact to voice		
−3	Moderate sedation	Any movement (but no eye contact) to voice		
−4	Deep sedation	No response to voice, but any movement to physical stimulation	Coma Unable to assess for delirium	
−5	Unarousable	No response to voice or physical stimulation		

Procedure
1. Observe patient. Is patient alert and calm (score 0)
   a. Does patient have behavior that is, consistent with restlessness or agitation (score +1 to +4 using the criteria listed above, under description)
2. If patient is not alert, in a loud speaking voice state patient's name and direct patient to open eyes and look at speaker. Repeat once if necessary. Can prompt patient to continue looking at speaker.
   a. Patient has eye opening and eye contact, which is sustained for more than 10 s (score 1).
   b. Patient has eye opening and eye contact, but this is not sustained for 10 s (score 2).
   c. Patient has any movement in response to voice, excluding eye contact (score 3).
3. If patient does not respond to voice, physically stimulate patient by shaking shoulder and then rubbing sternum if there is no response to shaking shoulder.
   a. Patient has any movement to physical stimulation (score 4).
   b. Patient has no response to voice or physical stimulation (score 5).

Abbreviation: LOC, level of consciousness.

Table 6
Riker Sedation–Agitation Scale (SAS)

Score	Term	Descriptor	Motor Subtype	LOC
7	Dangerous agitation	Pulling at ETT, trying to remove catheters, climbing over bedrail, striking at staff, thrashing side to side	Hyperactive	Altered
6	Very agitated	Requiring restraint and frequent verbal reminding of limits, biting ETT		
5	Agitated	Anxious or physically agitated, calms to verbal instructions		
4	Calm and cooperative	Calm, easily arousable, follows commands	—	Not altered
3	Sedated	Difficult to arouse but awakens to verbal stimuli or gentle shaking, follows simple commands but drifts off again	Hypoactive	Altered
2	Very sedated	Arouses to physical stimuli but does not communicate or follow commands, may move spontaneously		
1	Unarousable	Minimal or no response to noxious stimuli, does not communicate or follow commands	Unable to assess for delirium	

Procedure
1. Agitated patients are scored by their most severe degree of agitation as described
2. If patient is awake or awakens easily to voice ("awaken" means responds with voice or head shaking to a question or follows commands), that is, a SAS 4 (same as calm and appropriate – might even be napping).
3. If more stimuli such as shaking is required but patient eventually does awaken, that is, SAS 3.
4. If patient arouses to stronger physical stimuli (may be noxious) but never awakens to the point of responding yes/no or following commands, that is, a SAS of 2.
5. Little or no response to noxious physical stimuli represents a SAS of 1.
This helps to separate sedated patients into those you can eventually wake up (SAS 3), those you cannot awaken but can arouse (SAS 2), and those you cannot arouse (SAS 1).

Abbreviations: ETT, endotracheal tube; LOC, level of consciousness.
From Riker RR, Picard JT, Fraser GL. Prospective evaluation of the sedation-agitation scale for adult critically ill patients. Crit Care Med 1999;27(7):1327; with permission.

These tools are structured observational tools, and only require a few seconds to perform. Therefore, they should also be used with all routine assessments and as needed. Each of these tools are designed to quantify the patient's level of arousal. The current delirium screening tools were developed using the RASS, but the SAS has subsequently been validated for use in delirium.[19]

The RASS is scored between + 4 (combative) and −5 (unarousable or coma). For the majority of patients, the RASS goal will be 0. Scores above 0 (+1 to +4) represent an increased level of motor activity and hyperactivity. Scores below 0 (−1 to −3) indicate a decrease in arousal and therefore represent hypoactivity. Patients with a score of −4 (no response to voice, but does move to physical stimulation) or −5 (no response to voice or physical stimulation) are in coma, not able to be aroused, and are therefore unable to be assessed for delirium.

The SAS is used similarly. The scale is scored 1 to 7, with a score of 4 describing a patient who is calm, easily arousable, and follows commands. As with the RASS, if the SAS score is greater than 4 (5–7), the patient is hyperactive. If the SAS score is less than 4 (2–3), then the patient is hypoactive. If the score is 1, the patient is in coma and likewise unable to be assessed for delirium.

Step 4: Delirium Assessment

Delirium was first described by the ancient Greek, Celsus, in the first century A.D.[20] when he discussed the behavioral, attention, and cognition changes that he saw in his patients with fever or head trauma. The clinical assessment for delirium did not change much from his observational approach until the development of specific screening tools in the 20th Century. Most of these tools were developed for use in the outpatient setting, the hospital wards, and long-term care. Since that time, several tools have been developed specifically for use in the ICU. The 2 most widely used ICU tools were both first published in 2001: the Confusion Assessment Method for the ICU (CAM-ICU) and the Intensive Care Delirium Screening Checklist. These 2 tools are recommended for routine use in the ICU.[17,18]

The CAM-ICU was developed as an ICU-specific version of the existing tool, the Confusion Assessment Method (CAM). The CAM is a validated and widely used assessment tool. However, it was not designed for use in the ICU setting. A version of the CAM was developed specifically for use in the ICU setting. The resulting tool, the CAM-ICU (Appendix A) assesses for 4 items: acute or fluctuating alteration in mental status, inattentiveness, altered LOC, and disorganized thinking. If the patient has delirium, then she will be labeled "CAM +." To be CAM +, the patient must be arousable (RASS greater than −4 or SAS greater than 1) and be inattentive. In addition, she must also have at least one of the next 2 tested characteristics: altered LOC (RASS ≠ 4 or SAS ≠ 4), or disorganized thinking. The CAM-ICU has been validated with patients with acute ischemic stroke and intracerebral, but no other neuro ICU–specific patient populations.[21]

The second validated tool is the Intensive Care Delirium Screening Checklist (Appendix B). This 8-item tool assesses for delirium by evaluating LOC, attention, disorientation, hallucinations, hyperactivity or hypoactivity, inappropriate speech or mood, sleep/wake disturbance, and symptom fluctuation. To score the Intensive Care Delirium Screening Checklist, the clinician counts 1 point for every element of the tool that the patient is not able to perform correctly. If the score is 4 or greater, the patient has a positive delirium screen.

SUMMARY

This article has discussed what delirium is, the effects on patients and nurses, and patient vulnerabilities and triggers (risk factors), and outlined a comprehensive process for delirium monitoring. Appropriate, valid tools for pain, sedation–agitation, and delirium assessment and monitoring were reviewed. Because delirium is common, experienced by patients in every ICU setting, harmful to patients and nurses, and potentially preventable, the modern ICU nurse must be familiar with an evidence-based approach to monitoring every patient, with added vigilance for patients at high risk for delirium.

For more exploration of these topics, see Appendix C for a listing of additional resources.

REFERENCES

1. Case J, Khan S, Khalid R, et al. Epidemiology of acute kidney injury in the intensive care unit. Crit Care Res Pract 2013;2013:479730.
2. American Psychiatric Association. Diagnostic and statistical manual of mental disorders: DSM-5. Arlington (VA): American Psychiatric Association; 2013.
3. Meagher D, Moran M, Raju B, et al. A new data-based motor subtype schema for delirium. J Neuropsychiatry Clin Neurosci 2008;20(2):185–93.
4. Peterson JF, Pun BT, Dittus RS, et al. Delirium and its motoric subtypes: a study of 614 critically ill patients. J Am Geriatr Soc 2006;54(3):479–84.
5. Robinson TN, Raeburn CD, Tran ZV, et al. Motor subtypes of postoperative delirium in older adults. Arch Surg 2011;146(3):295–300.
6. Michaud CJ, Thomas WL, McAllen KJ. Early pharmacological treatment of delirium may reduce physical restraint use: a retrospective study. Ann Pharmacother 2014;48(3):328–34.
7. Bhalerao SU, Geurtjens C, Thomas GR, et al. Understanding the neuropsychiatric consequences associated with significant traumatic brain injury. Brain Inj 2013; 27(7–8):767–74.
8. Carin-Levy G, Mead GE, Nicol K, et al. Delirium in acute stroke: screening tools, incidence rates and predictors: a systematic review. J Neurol 2012;259(8): 1590–9.
9. Salluh JI, Wang H, Schneider EB, et al. Outcome of delirium in critically ill patients: systematic review and meta-analysis. BMJ 2015;350:h2538.
10. Heymann A, Radtke F, Schiemann A, et al. Delayed treatment of delirium increases mortality rate in intensive care unit patients. J Int Med Res 2010;38(5): 1584–95.
11. Anderson CP, Ngo LH, Marcantonio ER. Complications in postacute care are associated with persistent delirium. J Am Geriatr Soc 2012;60(6):1122–7.
12. Bélanger L, Ducharme F. Patients' and nurses' experiences of delirium: a review of qualitative studies. Nurs Crit Care 2011;16(6):303–15.
13. Maldonado JR. Neuropathogenesis of delirium: review of current etiologic theories and common pathways. Am J Geriatr Psychiatry 2013;21(12):1190–222.
14. van den Boogaard M, Pickkers P, Slooter AJ, et al. Development and validation of PRE-DELIRIC (PREdiction of DELIRium in ICu patients) delirium prediction model for intensive care patients: observational multicentre study. BMJ 2012; 344:e420.
15. van den Boogaard M, Schoonhoven L, Maseda E, et al. Recalibration of the delirium prediction model for ICU patients (PRE-DELIRIC): a multinational observational study. Intensive Care Med 2014;40(3):361–9.
16. Skrobik Y, Chanques G. The pain, agitation, and delirium practice guidelines for adult critically ill patients: a post-publication perspective. Ann Intensive Care 2013;3(1):9.
17. American Association of Critical-Care Nurses. AACN practice alert: assessing pain in the critically ill adult. 2013. Available at: http://www.aacn.org/WD/practice/docs/practicealerts/delirium-practice-alert-2011.pdf. Accessed August 20, 2015.
18. Barr J, Fraser GL, Puntillo K, et al. Clinical practice guidelines for the management of pain, agitation, and delirium in adult patients in the intensive care unit. Crit Care Med 2013;41(1):263–306.

19. Khan BA, Guzman O, Campbell NL, et al. Comparison and agreement between the Richmond Agitation-Sedation Scale and the Riker Sedation-Agitation Scale in evaluating patients' eligibility for delirium assessment in the ICU. Chest 2012; 142(1):48–54.

20. Adamis D, Treloar A, Martin FC, et al. A brief review of the history of delirium as a mental disorder. Hist Psychiatry 2007;18(4):459–69.

21. Mitasova A, Kostalova M, Bednarik J, et al. Post stroke delirium incidence and outcomes: validation of the confusion assessment method for the intensive care unit (CAM-ICU). Crit Care Med 2012;40(2):484–90.

22. Holly C, Cantwell ER, Jadotte Y. Acute delirium: differentiation and care. Crit Care Nurs Clin North Am 2012;24(1):131–47.

23. Zaal IJ, Devlin JW, Peelen LM, et al. A systematic review of risk factors for delirium in the ICU. Crit Care Med 2015;43(1):40–7.

24. Stites M. Observational pain scales in critically ill adults. Crit Care Nurse 2013; 33(3):68–78.

APPENDIX A

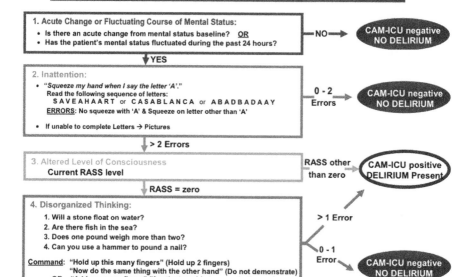

From Ely EW. Confusion Assessment Method for the ICU (CAM-ICU): The Complete Training Manual. Vanderbilt University. Available at: http://www.icudelirium.org/ docs/CAM_ICU_training.pdf. Copyright © 2002, E. Wesley Ely, MD, MPH and Vanderbilt University, all rights reserved.

APPENDIX B

Intensive Care Delirium Screening Checklist Worksheet (ICDSC)

- ☐ Score your patient over the entire shift. Components don't all need to be present at the same time.
- ☐ Components #1 through #4 require a focused bedside patient assessment. This cannot be completed when the patient is deeply sedated or comatose (i.e. RASS = -4 or -5).
- ☐ Components #5 through #8 are based on observations throughout the entire shift. Information from the prior 24 hrs. (i.e. from prior 1-2 nursing shifts) should be obtained for components #7 and #8.

		NO	0	1	YES
1. Altered Level of Consciousness					
Deep sedation/coma over entire shift (RASS = -4 or -5)	= UTA				
Normal wakefulness (RASS = 0) over the entire shift	= 0 points				
Light sedation (RASS= -1 to -3) **with sedation**	= 0 points				
Light sedation (RASS= -1 to -3) **with out sedation**	= 1 point				
Agitation (RASS = 1 to 4) at any point	= 1 point				

	NO	0	1	YES
2. Inattention				
Difficulty following instructions or conversation.				
Easily distracted by external stimuli.				
Will not reliably squeeze hands to spoken letter A:				
S A V E A H A A R T				

	NO	0	1	YES
3. Disorientation				
In addition to name, place, and date, does the patient recognize ICU caregivers?				
Does patient know what kind of place they are in?				

	NO	0	1	YES
4. Hallucination, delusion, or psychosis				
Ask the patient if they are having hallucinations or delusions.				
(e.g. trying to catch an object that isn't there).				
Are they afraid of the people or things around them?				

	NO	0	1	YES
5. Psychomotor agitation or retardation				
Either: a) Hyperactivity requiring the use of sedative drugs or restraints in order to control potentially dangerous behavior (e.g. pulling IV lines out or hitting staff)				
OR b) Hypoactive or clinically noticeable psychomotor slowing or retardation				

	NO	0	1	YES
6. Inappropriate speech or mood				
Patient displays: inappropriate emotion; disorganized or incoherent speech; sexual or inappropriate interactions; is either apathetic or overly demanding				

	NO	0	1	YES
7. Sleep-wake cycle disturbance				
Either: frequent awakening/< 4 hours sleep at night OR sleeping during much of the day				

	NO	0	1	YES
8. Symptom Fluctuation				
Fluctuation of any of the above symptoms over a 24 hr. period.				

TOTAL SHIFT SCORE: _____
(0 – 8)

Score	Classification
0	Normal
1 – 3	Subsyndromal Delirium
4 - 8	Delirium

Adapted from Bergeron N, Dubois MJ, Dumont M, et al. Intensive care delirium screening checklist: evaluation of a new screening tool. Intensive Care Med 2001;27(5):862; with permission.

APPENDIX C

Additional delirium resources

Guidelines
- Clinical Practice Guidelines for the Management of Pain, Agitation, and Delirium in Adult Patients in the Intensive Care Unit[18]
  - Available at: http://www.learnicu.org/SiteCollectionDocuments/Pain,%20Agitation,%20Delirium.pdf
- Delirium—diagnosis, prevention and management: NICE Clinical Guideline 103. (NICE, 2010)
  - Available at: guidance.nice.org.uk/cg103
- American Association of Critical-Care Nurses (AANC) Practice Alert: Delirium assessment and management (American Association of Critical-Care Nurses, 2011)
  - Available at: http://www.aacn.org/WD/practice/docs/practicealerts/delirium-practice-alert-2011.pdf

Web Sites
- Agency for Healthcare Research and Quality, Patient Safety Net (AHRQ, PSNet)
  - U.S. Department of Health and Human Services
  - Searchable database of current guidelines and supporting evidence
  - Available at: http://www.ahrq.gov
- Agency for Healthcare Research and Quality, Patient Safety Net (AHRQ, PSNet)
  - U.S. Department of Health and Human Services
  - Searchable database of multiple patient safety resources related to delirium
  - Available at: https://psnet.ahrq.gov
- ICU Delirium
  - Sponsored by Vanderbilt University Medical Center, Nashville, Tennessee
  - Excellent source of Medical Provider and Patient/Family resources
  - Available at: http://www.icudelirium.org
- ICU Liberation Campaign
  - Sponsored by the Society for Critical Care Medicine
  - Established to educate medical professionals and to provide tools to treat and prevent pain, agitation, and delirium in the ICU
  - Available at: http://www.iculiberation.org

Abbreviations: ICU, intensive care unit; NIC, National Institute for Health and Care Excellence.

Neuroradiology of the Brain

Susan Yeager, MS, RN, CCRN, ACNP-BC, FNCS

KEYWORDS

- Brain imaging • Neuroradiology • Brain diagnostics

KEY POINTS

- Neurologic imaging has brought intracranial structures from being a "dark continent" into the light; through technologic advances, what once took days to obtain can now be completed in a matter of minutes.
- Single-plane images can now be obtained in multiple visual planes providing increased information and at times 3-D information on brain pathology or anatomic structures.
- The wide availability of many of these techniques, with varying costs and times for acquisition, presents several options when practitioners look to answer questions regarding differential diagnosis.
- When to use which radiographic technique varies by diagnosis but often requires an overlap of the repertoire to achieve the information desired.
- Ongoing study and evolution of techniques must be focused on the optimization, standardization, and clinical validation of how this technology can ultimately have an impact on care of cerebral pathology.

INTRODUCTION

A variety of imaging modalities are currently used to evaluate the brain. Prior to the 1970s, however, neurologic imaging primarily involved radiographs, invasive procedures for spinal and carotid artery air and contrast injection, and painful patient manipulation to gather information on brain pathology. In 1895, Röntgen discovered x-ray imaging but it was years before neurologic application was realized. This was because at that time the brain was considered inaccessible to imaging and referred to as "the dark continent."[1] Through the ensuing years, neuroradiology was slow to be explored. During World War I, plain radiography was used primitively in some centers. In 1918, ventriculography was discovered with encephalography soon to follow. Images were obtained through the procedure of air mylography. Using this technique, air was

The author has no disclosures.
The Ohio State University Wexner Medical Center, College of Nursing, The Ohio State University, Neurocritical Care Graves Hall, 333 West 10th Avenue, Suite 3172, Columbus, OH 43210, USA
E-mail address: syeager@columbus.rr.com

injected into cerebrospinal fluid (CSF) and/or carotid vessels with the intention of high-lighting the presence of hydrocephalus or the localization of tumors. The year 1925 came with the discovery of contrast agent injection (Lipiodol). In 1931, after years of experimentation, Moniz described contrast-enhanced arteriography as a means to further highlight brain structures. Acceptance was slow (in part due to the method of cut down exposure of the carotid arteries with subsequent scarring). In 1944, however, the concept was revisited by Engeset and arteriography became a universally accepted technique. World War II spurred the use of radioactive substance instillation to assist with tumor localization. Geiger counters were used as an external tool for tumor detection. This was due to the tumor's increased uptake of radioactive agents. A Wood lamp was also used after brain exposure to highlight the differences in hue of normal and tumorous tissue under ultraviolet light (normal brain was grayish and gliomas appeared yellow). The 1960s was an era when commercial manufacturers began work to perfect scanning devices.[1] Since that time, exciting advances in neuroradiology have moved the brain from being a dark continent that was "mute to x-rays" to evaluation techniques that illuminate brain contents and pathology. These advances, when used properly, enable quick acquisition of images to enable prompt diagnosis and treatment of various disease entities. For the purposes of this article, anatomy, diagnostic principles, and clinical application of brain imaging beyond plain radiographs are reviewed.

ANATOMY OVERVIEW
Tissue

To better understand what the various imaging techniques reflect, a basic overview of normal brain structures is necessary. Intricate knowledge of all anatomy is not necessary but basic knowledge is important. The brain is divided into 3 major areas: the cerebrum, the brainstem, and the cerebellum. The cerebrum is comprised of the frontal, parietal, and occipital lobes (**Fig. 1**). It is composed of both cerebral hemispheres,

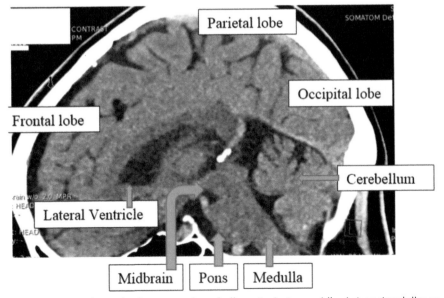

Fig. 1. Tissue: cerebrum, brainstem, and cerebellum. Brainstem: midbrain/pons/medulla; cerebrum: frontal/parietal/occipital lobes.

thalamus and hypothalamus, and basal ganglia. The brainstem is composed of the midbrain, pons, and medulla. The cerebellum is located inferior and posterior to the cerebrum and brainstem (**Fig. 2**).[2] Important landmarks include the central sulcus, which separates the frontal and parietal lobes; the sylvian fissure, which divides the frontal and parietal lobes from the temporal lobe; and the parieto-occipital sulcus, which separates the parietal and occipital lobes and the preoccipital notch that separates the occipital lobe from the cerebellum (**Fig. 3**).[3]

Arterial Vasculature

The cerebrovascular circulation consists of an intricate maze of vessels that provide oxygen-rich blood to the brain. It consists of the anterior (carotid portion) and the posterior (vertebrobasilar portion) sections. The anterior circulation refers to the common carotids and their distal branches, including the internal carotid arteries, the middle cerebral arteries, and the anterior cerebral arteries (**Fig. 4**). The posterior circulation refers to the vertebral arteries, the basilar artery, and the posterior arteries. Blood travels into the system through 2 vertebral arteries and 2 internal carotid arteries (**Fig. 5**). Blood then empties into the circle of Willis, located at the base of the skull. This is a circulatory anastomosis that provides blood to the brain and surrounding structures. The entire circle is made up of the basilar artery, the bilateral posterior cerebral arteries, the bilateral posterior communicating arteries, the bilateral internal carotid arteries, the anterior communicating arteries, and the bilateral anterior cerebral arteries. The middle cerebral arteries are not considered a part of the circle but are important vessels in the brain's blood supply (**Fig. 6**).[2]

Venous Drainage

Once blood has entered the cerebrovascular system, it traverses back to the heart through the venous drainage system. The normal venous outflow process progresses through the paired internal cerebral veins and basal veins of Rosenthal, which come together to form the vein of Galen. The vein of Galen is then joined by the sagittal sinus, which lies along the edge of the falx to form the straight sinus. This sinus drains to the

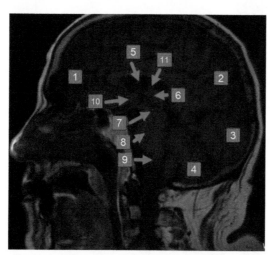

Fig. 2. Tissue cerebral hemispheres: thalamus, hypothalamus, and basal ganglia. 1, Frontal lobe; 2, parietal lobe; 3, occipital lobe; 4, cerebellum; 5, CSF-filled lateral ventricle; 6, thalmus; 7, midbrain; 8, pons; 9, medulla; 10, hypothalmus; and 11, basal ganglia.

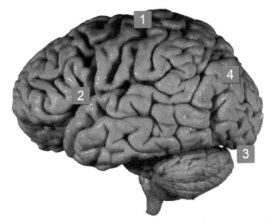

Fig. 3. Brain anatomic fissures, notch, and sulcus. 1, Central sulcus; 2, sylvian fissure; 3, pre-occipital notch; and 4, parieto-occipital sulcus.

confluence of sinuses. Superficial cerebral veins join to form the superior sagittal sinus, which also drains into the confluences of sinuses to the sigmoid sinus, to the jugular bulb, and into the internal jugular veins (**Fig. 7**).[3]

Ventricular System

In addition to the vascular components providing blood to and draining blood from the brain, there is a ventricular system within the brain. This closed ventricular system provides a conduit for CSF, which is continuously produced within the brain. This system consists of the following. There are 2 lateral ventricles, 1 on either side of midline

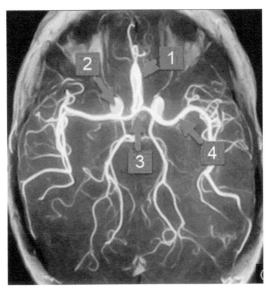

Fig. 4. Arterial vasculature anterior circulation. 1, Anterior cerebral arteries; 2, carotid artery; 3, anterior communicating artery; and 4, middle cerebral artery.

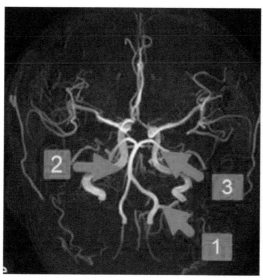

Fig. 5. Arterial vasculature posterior circulation. 1, Vertebral artery; 2, basilar artery; and 3, posterior cerebral artery.

located at the lower and inner parts of the cerebral hemispheres. Each lateral ventricle has 3 horns. The anterior horn curves forward into the frontal lobe. The posterior horn curves backwards and inward toward the occipital lobe. The lateral horn descends into the temporal lobe. Flow from the lateral ventricle traverses through the foramina of Monro. The third ventricle is a midline inner brain structure. The third ventricle drains fluid through the cerebral aqueduct or aqueduct of Sylvius into the fourth ventricle.

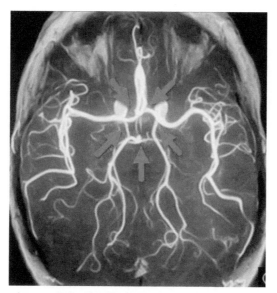

Fig. 6. Arterial vasculature: circle of Willis (*arrows*).

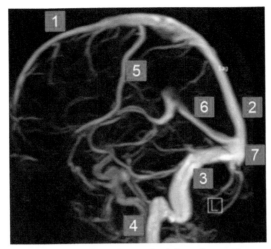

Fig. 7. Major venous vasculature. 1, Superior sagittal sinus; 2, superior sagittal sinus; 3, transverse sinus; 4, internal jugular vein; 5, superior vein of Trolard; 6, straight sinus; and 7, confluence of sinuses.

From the fourth ventricle, the CSF circulates through the lateral foramina of Luschka and through the midline foramen of Magendie into the cisternal magnum. From this point, the fluid enters into the subarachnoid space (**Fig. 8**).[2]

DEFINITIONS

After becoming familiar with neurologic anatomy, the next step in neuroradiographic learning is to become familiar with definitions of commonly used terms. These terms are standardized, which translates to a shared understanding between providers when verbal descriptors are used. Common terms that are used during radiographic interpretation are explained.

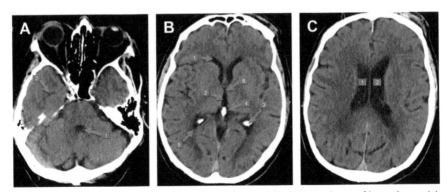

Fig. 8. Ventricular system: temporal horn, fourth ventricle, anterior horn of lateral ventricle, third ventricle, choroid plexus, pineal gland, posterior/occipital horn of lateral ventricle, foramen of Monro, and lateral ventricles. (*A*) Brain base section. 1, Fourth ventricle, and 2, temporal horn. (*B*) Central brain section. 1, Anterior horn of lateral ventricle; 2, third ventricle; 3, choroid plexus; 4, pineal gland; 5, posterior/occipital horn of lateral ventricle; and 6, foramen of Monro. (*C*) Upper brain section. 1 And 2, lateral ventricles.

Key to radiograph interpretation is a basic understanding of neuroradiographic concepts. Prior to the 1960s to 1970s, diagnostic neuroradiology was described as a study of shadows.[1] With advances in techniques, shadows became focused through a display of shades of white, black, and gray.[4] In general, the variation of shade is reflective of the density of the object. If an object is more dense, fewer x-ray beams pass through it. For example, air is not dense and, therefore, enables a large number of radiographic beams to pass through. Thus, air shows up as black on an image. Alternately, bone is dense and presents as white. These basic rules do not always apply when certain MRI techniques are used. (See **Fig. 9** for a depiction of gray-scale representations of radiographic images.) Depending on the gray-scale representation, hypodescriptors or hyperdescriptors can be used to describe images noted when reviewing an examination.

- Gray scale—This term is a representation of intensities of radiographic structures reflected in shades of gray (see **Fig. 9**; **Table 1**).
- Hypointensity/hyperintensity—These are MRI terms used to describe structures that are low areas on the gray scale (hypointense/dark) or high areas of uptake on the gray scale (hyperintense/white).
- Hypodensity/hyperdensity—CT scan terms used to describe structures that are low areas on the gray scale (hypodense/dark) or high areas of uptake on the gray scale (hyperdense/white).

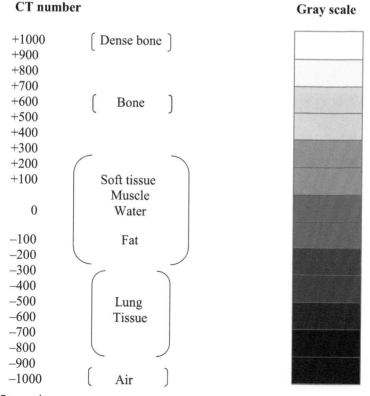

Fig. 9. Gray scale.

Table 1 MRI/CT gray scale summary			
Normal Tissue	T1	T2	CT
Dense bone	Dark	Dark	Bright
Air	Dark	Dark	Dark
Fat	Bright	Less bright	Dark
Water	Dark	Bright	Dark
Brain	Anatomic	Intermediate	Intermediate

The axis in which an image is captured is also important when interpreting and describing what is seen. The common planes of image acquisition are defined.

- Axial—An imaging plane that is a transverse plane perpendicular to the long axis of the body (**Fig. 10**)
- Sagittal—An imaging plane that is a longitudinal plane that divides the body into right and left sections (**Fig. 11**)
- Coronal—An imaging plane that is a slice or section made that cuts across the body from one side to the other (front to back) (**Fig. 12**)

In addition to understanding the plane of the image, a basic knowledge of imaging techniques is necessary to understand and be able to articulate what is being viewed. Some of these terms are descriptions of a physics technique regarding how the body is manipulated to get the image desired. Some of the other terms are used to reflect specific regions of the brain.

- Noncontrasted images—These are images obtained without the use of contrast mediums.

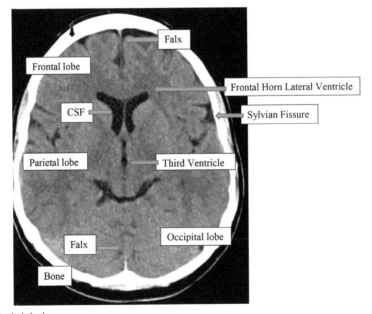

Fig. 10. Axial plane.

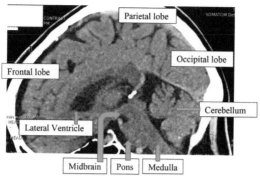

Fig. 11. Sagittal plane.

- Contrast images—These are images obtained with the use of contrast mediums. Contrast is used to facilitate visualization of suspected neoplasms or brain infections. In CT scan imaging, contrast material contains iodine, which is denser than brain or broken-down blood-brain barriers (**Table 2**).[5]
- Contrast medium/agent—Contrast is a radiopaque substance used in radiography to permit visualization of body structures.
- Gray matter—Anatomic areas of the nervous system where the nerve fibers are unmyelinated. It contains the cell body and dendrites of the nerve cells, that is, the cerebral cortex.
- White matter—Anatomic areas of the nervous system where the myelinated axons occur
- Radiofrequency (RF) pulse—MRI technique where short electromagnetic signals oscillate to change the direction of the magnetic field. They are cycled at a rate of pulses per second.
- Relaxation time—This is the time it takes protons to regain their equilibrium state during MRI. T1 and T2 are 2 types of relaxation phases.

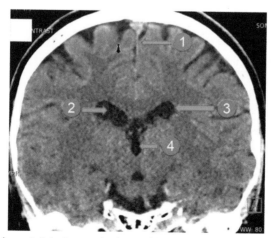

Fig. 12. Coronal plane. 1, Falx; 2, anterior horn of lateral ventricle; 3, lateral ventricle; and 4, third ventricle.

Table 2
MRI with gadolinium enhancement

Potential Diagnosis Evaluated	
Lymphoma	Toxoplasmosis
Tuberculosis	Glioblastoma multiform
Inflammation	Histoplasmosis
Bacterial abscess	Demyelination (active)
Radiation necrosis	Necrotic metastatic disease
Coccidiomycosis	Actinomycosis
Nocardia	Blastopmycosis
Whipple	Listeria
Bartonella	Cystercercosis

- T1—This is the time it takes for 63% of longitudinal (parallel to the magnetic field) relaxation of protons to occur. Not all tissues get back to equilibrium equally quickly, and a tissue's T1 reflects the amount of time its protons' spins realign with the main magnetic field. Fat quickly realigns its longitudinal magnetization, and it therefore appears bright on a T1-weighted image. Conversely, water has a much slower longitudinal magnetization realignment after an RF pulse (RFP). Thus, water has low signal and appears dark. T1 is considered the anatomic image. Clues to recognizing T1: CSF is black, subcutaneous fat is white (**Box 1, Fig. 13**).
- T2—This is the time it takes for 63% of transverse (perpendicular) relaxation of protons to occur during MRI acquisition. Not all tissues get back to equilibrium equally quickly. Water is white on T2 imaging. T2 is considered the pathologic image. Most pathology shows up as high signal (bright), including surrounding edema (**Box 2, Fig. 14**).
- T2 fluid-attenuated inversion recovery (FLAIR)—This sequence is basically a T2 image without the CSF brightness. The CSF is nulled out (appears black). In

Box 1
T1 characteristics (see Fig. 13)

White matter is brighter than gray matter

Dark (hypointense)
- CSF
- Increased water–edema, tumor, infarct, inflammation, infection, hemorrhage (hyperacute or chronic)
- Low proton density–calcification
- Flow void

Bright (hyperintense)
- Fat
- Subacute hemorrhage
- Melanin
- Protein-rich fluid
- Slow-flowing blood
- Gadolinium
- Laminar necrosis of an infarct

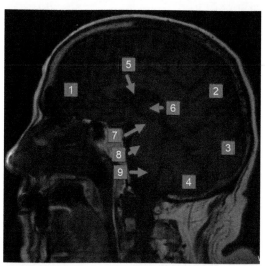

Fig. 13. MRI T1. 1, Frontal lobe; 2, parietal lobe; 3, occipital lobe; 4, cerebellum; 5, CSF–filled lateral ventricle; 6, thalmus; 7, midbrain; 8, pons; and 9, medulla.

this recovery period, water is reduced by timing the delay of the inversion pulse. In this phase, CSF is gray rather than the white seen on normal T2 imaging. This technique attempts to minimize distraction of the CSF brightness while highlighting underlying pathology (**Fig. 15**).

- Diffusion-weighted imaging (DWI)—Follows the changes in the movement of water through tissues and uses these changes as a contrast medium. Free diffusion of protons occurs only when cell membrane integrity is lost. Therefore, this MRI sequencing is sensitive to abnormal water motion and diffusion through the tissues. DWI is a manipulated T2 image and, therefore, high signal areas can be caused by T2 shine-through. DWI is used in acute stroke identification[6] as well as to differentiate abscess versus necrosis versus cystic brain lesions[7] (**Fig. 16**).
- T2 shine-through—Term used when on a DWI a structure is bright. Because DWIs are based on a T2 image, anything that is bright on T2 can also be bright on DWI. Rule: high-signal DWI (bright) and low-signal ADC (dark) = true abnormality; high-signal DWI (bright) and high-signal ADC (bright) = false positive for an abnormality.

Box 2
T2 characteristics (see Fig. 14)

Gray matter is brighter than white matter.

Dark (hypointense)
- Low proton density, calcification, fibrous tissue
- Deoxyhemoglobin, methemoglobin (intracellular), iron, hemosiderin, melanin
- Protein-rich fluid
- Flow void

Bright (hyperintense)
- Increased water–edema, tumor, infarct, inflammation, infection, subdural collection
- Methemoglobin (extracellular) in subacute hemorrhage

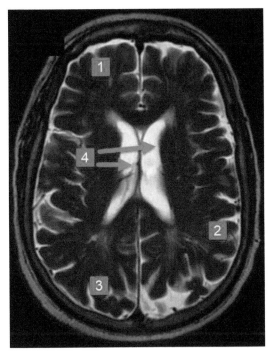

Fig. 14. MRI T2. 1, Frontal lobe; 2, parietal lobe; 3, occipital lobe; and 4, CSF-filled lateral ventricles.

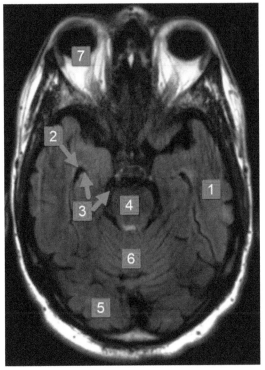

Fig. 15. MRI T2 FLAIR. 1, Temporal lobe; 2, temporal horn of lateral ventricle; 3, nulled out CSF; 4, pons; 5, occipital lobe; 6, cerebellum; and 7, eyeball.

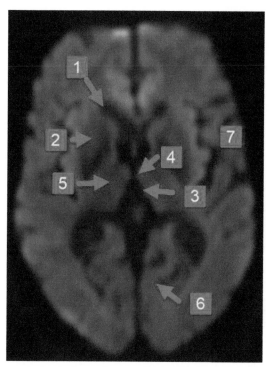

Fig. 16. Normal MRI DWI. 1, Anterior horn lateral ventricle; 2, external capsule; 3, third ventricle; 4, foramen of Monro; 5, thalmus; 6, occipital horn of lateral ventricle; and 7, insula.

- Apparent diffusion coefficient (ADC)—This is a measure of the magnitude of diffusion (of water molecules) within tissue and is commonly clinically calculated using MRI with DWI. ADC values are calculated automatically by the software and then displayed as a parametric map that reflects the degree of diffusion of water molecules through different tissues. The extent of tissue cellularity and the presence of intact cell membranes help determine the impedance of water molecule diffusion. This impedance of water molecule diffusion can be quantitatively assessed using the ADC value. ADC maps are devoid of T2 effects that may mimic or obscure lesions on DWI (**Fig. 17**).[8,9]
- Susceptibility-weighted imaging (SWI)—An echo MRI sequence that is particularly sensitive to compounds, which distort the local magnetic field and as such make it useful in detecting blood products, calcium, and so forth. The most common use of SWI is for the identification of small amounts of hemorrhage/blood product or calcium, which may or may not be apparent on other MRI sequences. Blood is dark in this sequence (**Fig. 18**).
- Perfusion-weighted imaging (PWI)—Radioisotopic imaging that uses the difference in blood flow through organs as a means of diagnosing diseases, such as stroke or malignancies (**Fig. 19**).
- Diffusion-perfusion mismatch—Indicates a deficit on PWI, which exceeds the zone of diffusion on DWIs. Differences on diffusion to perfusion reflect salvageable brain tissue that is at risk for infarction.
- Cerebral blood flow (CBF)—Term applied to MRI or CT perfusion (CTP) scan. This is defined as the volume of blood moving through a given volume of brain

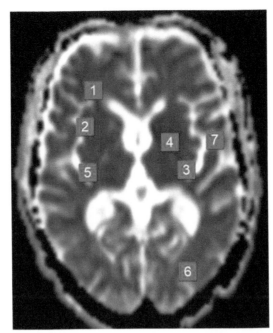

Fig. 17. Normal MRI ADC with contrast. 1, Anterior horn lateral ventricle; 2, external capsule; 3, third ventricle; 4, foramen of Monro; 5, thalmus; 6, occipital horn of lateral ventricle; and 7, insula.

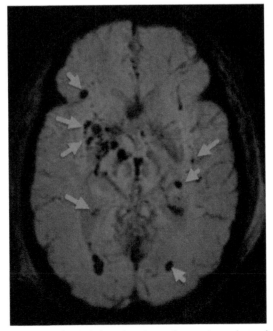

Fig. 18. MRI SWI of traumatic brain injured patient after motorcycle crash. Red arrows, multiple microhemorrhages scattered throughout brain parenchyma.

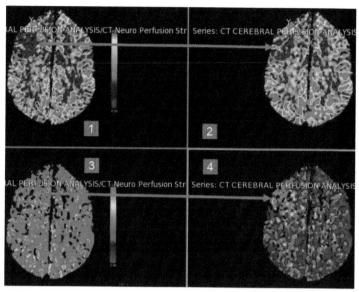

Fig. 19. Redemonstration of matched right frontal middle cerebral artery ischemic stroke. 1, CBF; 2, CBV; 3, MTT; and 4, TTD.

per unit time. CBF has units of milliliters of blood per 100 g of brain tissue per minute. Blood flow in stroke is usually prolonged but not always making time to peak (TTP) more sensitive.[10]

- Cerebral blood volume (CBV)—Term applied to MRI or CTP imaging. It is the total volume of contrast in a given unit volume of the brain. This includes contrast in the tissues as well as blood in the large capacitance vessels, such as arteries, arterioles, capillaries, venules, and veins. CBV has units of milliliters of blood per 100 g of brain tissue. CBV may initially be low in an occluded or narrowed vessel. Low CBV is bad and indicative of low flow states (ie, stroke).[6,10]
- Mean transit time (MTT)—Term applied to MRI or CTP scans. This is defined as the average transit time of blood traversing through a given brain region. This transit time of blood varies depending on the distance traveled between arterial inflow and venous outflow. It also varies with impedance of blood flow. Mathematically, MTT is related to both CBV and CBF. MTT = CBV/CBF.[6]
- TTP—term applied to MRI or CTP scans. This is defined as the time it takes for contrast to flow into a specific area of the brain. The peak is the top of the calculated curve created as the contrast infuses into an area. This is a sensitive tool for determining decreased contrast flow because blood going through collateral or narrowed vessels increases the TTP in stroke patients.[8,10,11]

BASIC BRAIN IMAGING
Computerized Tomography Scan: Brain

The conceptualization of the CT scan dates back to 1917. The foundation lay in mathematical theories conceived by an Austrian mathematician named Johann Radon. Later, Polish mathematician Stefan Kaczmarz made additional mathematical discoveries that, in turn, were later adapted by Hounsfield for use in the CT scanner. Sir Godfrey Hounsfield, working at EMI Laboratories, first conceived of the idea of CT scan imaging in 1967. It began with him thinking that what was inside a box could be determined if radiographs were taken from every angle of the outside. At the same time, McLeod Cormack was also manipulating mathematical principles behind CT. Both men were credited for the discovery. The first prototype was finished in 1971 and was only designed to scan the head. It was first tested on a preserved brain followed by imaging of a fresh cow's brain from the local butcher before Hounsfield used it on himself. With the concept proved, CT was moved to an actual patient. In 1971 it was performed on a patient suffering with a cerebral cyst. The prototype took several hours to get the data required to scan a single slice and required several days to compile the information into a single image. The images it made were crude by today's standards but were the first that allowed physicians to see soft tissue structures by imaging.[12]

Atkinson Morley Hospital in Wimbledon, London, was the site of the first commercial CT scanner. The first to be installed in the United States were at the Massachusetts General Hospital and the Mayo Clinic. The first US scan occurred on June 19, 1973, but it took a few years to gain widespread popularity. As the diagnostic application became known, CT scans became in high demand. Today, there are approximately 6000 CT scanners in use, with image acquisition occurring in minutes versus days. Expansion of this imaging's building blocks has progressed to applications that now include vascular and perfusion CT scan technology.[12]

Physics

Tomography stems from the Greek *tomos*, meaning section. CT imaging was developed directly from conventional x-ray technology. Like conventional radiographs, CT scans measure the density of studied tissues. The difference from conventional radiograph is that rather than taking 1 view, the x-ray beam is rotated around the patient to take many different views of a single slice of a patient's brain. Once obtained, the images are reconstructed by the computer to reflect detailed images of all the structures included in the slice, such as air, bone, liquid, and soft tissue. To obtain the image, the patient lies on a table that moves the patient's body in small steps through a doughnut-shaped scanner. With each step of the table, a thin x-ray beam is scanned through the patient at many different angles and picked up by detectors on the opposite side of the ring. As the beam passes through the patient, the radiographs are partially absorbed by the tissue it encounters. The amount of energy absorbed depends on the density of the tissue traversed. Calculations from the information obtained from the multiple detectors lining the inside of the ring are translated to calculate the densities at every point within the horizontal slice. This information is then translated to reflect an image. As the technology has advanced, multiple slices can now be acquired simultaneously. Spiral (helical) CT can acquire data continuously without stops, similarly to peeling an apple skin off the core all in 1 section. This technology reduces radiation exposure as well as increasing the resolution and speed of image acquisition.[5]

Images obtained are displayed with different densities. Dense structures, like bone or calcifications, appear white on images. Less dense material, such as air, appear black. CT density is often expressed in different Hounsfield units (HU). The HU scale is based on the following: bone = 2000, water = 0, and air = −1000 (see **Fig. 9**).

Advantages/disadvantages

The potential advantages and disadvantages of CT imaging are summarized.

Advantages

- The major advantage is the widespread availability, relatively low cost, and rapid acquisition time.

- CT is the only available modality for evaluation in patients with contraindications to MRI scanning or when screening for MRI cannot be obtained.
- Open set-up of equipment creates ease of patient placement while alleviating the potential of claustrophobia.

Disadvantages

- Uses ionizing radiation
- Radiation dose is additive, so the more images obtained, the higher the dose of radiation to which a patient is exposed.
- CT angiography (CTA) and CTP image processing is more labor intensive than magnetic resonance angiography (MRA) and magnetic resonance perfusion (MRP).
- Iodinated IV contrast is required for CT with contrast, CTA, CTP, and CT venogram imaging that could have an impact on kidney function or may not be possible due to a patient's kidney function.
- Contrast allergies may exist.
- Screening for contrast allergies or renal disease may be difficult in an acute setting.
- Posterior structures are not as well visualized due to bone artifact.[6]

MRI: Brain

MRI is an imaging modality that uses nonionizing radiation to create diagnostic useful images. The development of MRI techniques is a new phenomenon. The concept of MRI was first described by Felix Bloch and Edward Purcell in 1946. It was initially called nuclear MRI after its early use for chemical analysis. The nuclear description was eventually dropped given the misconception by patients regarding the potential nuclear radiation that would be received from the study. It was not until 1971 when the potential medical uses of this technology were realized. This occurred when Damadian discovered that magnetic relaxation times differed between tissue and tumor. In 1975, Ernst formed the basis of current MRI techniques when he proposed phase and frequency encoding and Fourier transform. Charles Dumoulin developed MRA in 1987 and functional MRI was established in 1993.[13]

Physics

The physics behind MRI is more complicated than for CT. A basic understanding of these physics is necessary, however, to understand the process of image acquisition. A high-level overview of these processes is provided.

A MRI scanner consists of a large and very strong magnet in which the patient lies. A radio wave antenna is then used to send signals to the body, which then receives signals back. These returning signals are then converted into images by a computer attached to the scanner.[13]

The principles of MRI surround the absorption and emission of RF energy without ionizing radiation. After being placed on the imaging table and positioned within the MRI cylinder, a static magnetic field is applied. Hydrogen protons within the patient's body align to this magnetic field. Throughout this magnetification process, a RFP is emitted from the scanner. The magnification and pulse waves are tuned to a specific range of frequencies at which hydrogen protons react (usually 0.3T–1.5T). This proton reaction results in some of the hydrogen protons being "knocked" 180° out of alignment with the static magnetic field and being forced into phase with other hydrogen protons. As the energy from the RFP is dissipated, the hydrogen protons return to baseline alignment within the static magnetic field. During this realignment, an emitted

RF is created. The MRI signal is derived from the hydrogen protons as they move back into alignment with the magnetic field and fall out of phase with each other. T1 relaxation and T2 decay images are obtained from this initial magnetic field alteration. The MRI signal is then broken down and spatially located to produce images.

Spatial encoding of the MRI signal is accomplished through the use of gradients (smaller magnetic fields). The gradients are turned on and off quickly, causing vibration of the protons, which perturb the main magnetic field. This causes hydrogen protons in different locations to respond at slightly different rates, which results in image variation. Images obtained during the standard examination vary from facility to facility and examination times fluctuate depending on the sequencing and anatomic location obtained.[13]

Diffusion-Weighted Imaging: Brain

DWI was first described in 1965 by Stejskal and Tanner but it was not until the mid-1980s that DWI routinely became available. DWI has proved highly sensitive to the early identification of ischemic tissue injury (even before conventional MRIs) and normal and abnormal microstructural brain tissues.

Physics

DWI is a result of differences in the magnitude of diffusion of water molecules within the brain. The higher the degree of random motion, the more the magnetic resonance signal is lost. Conversely, the lower the degree of random motion, the less the magnetic resonance signal is lost. DWIs are partially T2 and partially diffusion weighted. This is because T2 signal intensity is decreased by an amount of magnetic resonance signal loss determined by diffusion. Applied clinically, DWI has proved to show tissue injury within 30 minutes of vessel occlusion, before conventional T1-weighted or T2-weighted sequences show pathology. DWI is especially useful in the identification of acute stroke. By combining DWI with perfusion-weighted images, matching results can indicate oligemic tissue or a penumbra tissue at risk for infarct evolution. Through early recognition, treatment strategies can be initiated quicker to minimize tissue effected.[9]

Advantages/disadvantages

Advantages There are several advantages to MRI over other neurodiagnostic studies. These advantages include

- The ability to image without the use of ionizing radiation (x-ray and CT scanning)
- Images may be acquired in multiple planes (axial, sagittal, coronal, or oblique) without repositioning the patient. CT images have only recently been able to be reconstructed in multiple planes with the same spatial resolution.
- MRI demonstrates superior soft tissue contrast over CT scans and plain films, making it the ideal examination of the brain, spine, joints, and other soft tissue body parts.
- Some angiographic images can be obtained without the use of contrast material, unlike CT or conventional angiography.
- Advanced techniques, such as diffusion and perfusion, allow for specific tissue characterization rather than merely macroscopic imaging.
- Functional MRI allows visualization of both active parts of the brain during certain activities and understanding of the underlying networks.
- The ability to visualize posterior structures of the brain better than CT imaging

Disadvantages There are several disadvantages and challenges to implementing MRI scanning. These disadvantages include

- MRI scans are more expensive than CT scans and take longer to acquire so patient comfort is sometimes an issue. Additionally, images are subject to unique artifacts that must be recognized and abated.
- MRI scanning is not safe for patients with some metal implants and foreign bodies. Careful attention to safety measures is necessary to avoid serious injury to patients and staff. This requires special MRI-compatible equipment and stringent adherence to safety protocols.
- Claustrophobia and patient size may preclude the ability to obtain images.
- Length of an examination and decreased visualization of the patient throughout an examination can put certain patients at risk for clinical decompensation (**Table 3**).[6]

ADVANCED COMPUTERIZED TOMOGRAPHY/MRI/ANGIOGRAPHY IMAGING: VASCULAR
Computerized Tomography Angiography: Brain/Neck

The concept of visualizing brain and neck arterial systems via CT was introduced by Heinz and others in the 1984. Actualization of this imaging modality into practice was only recently achieved due to recent technological advances.[14]

Table 3
CT scan versus MRI—clinical situations

Clinical Situation	CT Scan Better	MRI Scan Better
Head trauma	★	
Acute brain hemorrhage	★	
Old brain hemorrhage		★
Infection		★
Brain lesion		★
Ischemic stroke		★
Brainstem lesion		★
Skull fracture	★	
Tissue anatomic detail		★
Vascular anatomic detail	★	
Cost	★	
Speed of acquisition	★	
Availability	★	
Patient comfort	★[a]	
Metallic substance within the body	★	
Renal impairment		★
Radiation exposure		★

[a] Open MRI scanners and large-bore bariatric scanners are now available in some facilities to help minimize patient discomfort.

Physics

Computerized tomography angiography CTA is a method of rapid injection of iodine-rich intravenous (IV) contrast. This contrast is used in combination with helical CT scan techniques to rapidly obtain images of the cerebral and neck vessels to evaluate the presence of stenosis, occlusion, vasospasm, and dissection. These images are reconstructed into 3-D views through computer mathematical calculations. Although each CT vendor offers slightly different techniques, several basics apply to all. The scan of the neck begins at the aortic arch and extends to the skull base or 1 cm above the dorsum sellae if intracranial information is desired. CTA of the brain begins at C2 and extends to the vertex. CTA is highly accurate. Using conventional angiography as the comparison, the specificity and sensitivity of CTA are 98.1% and 98.4%, respectively.

Magnetic resonance angiography

Contrast MRA uses MRI technology to evaluate cerebral vessels for the presence of occlusion, dissection, aneurysm, functional areas of the brain, and vasospasm (**Fig. 20**). A variety of techniques can be used to obtain vessel imaging. The most common method is based on the injection of contrast material (generally gadolinium) through IV access. Phase contrast MRA images evaluates blood flow velocity. Using this method, contrast is injected in the vein with precontrast and during the first pass of the agent images obtained. Subtracting these 2 images only shows blood vessels while blocking out surrounding tissue. Contrast injection shortens the acquisition of T1 image of blood versus all other tissues (except fat), resulting in bright images of blood. Because this technique is 4 times slower than time of flight (TOF), it is useful in differentiating slow versus absent flow because it detects only truly patent

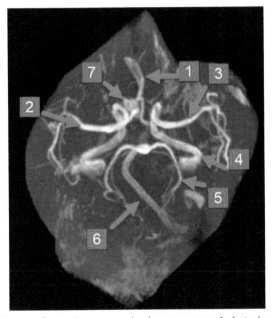

Fig. 20. MRA 3-D image of anterior communicating aneurysm. 1, Anterior cerebral artery; 2, middle cerebral artery; 3, middle cerebral artery; 4, internal carotid artery; 5, posterior cerebral artery; 6, basilar artery; and 7, anterior communicating artery aneurysm.

vessels.[15] Many other techniques for performing MRA exist and can be classified into 2 general groups: flow-dependent methods and flow-independent methods.

Flow dependent The most commonly used flow-dependent example of MRA imaging is TOF. TOF uses a short echo time, which limits the number of excitation pulses, which means the blood is not saturated, giving it a much higher signal (bright) than the saturated stationary tissue. This method is dependent on flowing blood against surrounding tissue recognizing that blood has greater proton density than stationary tissue. Because this imaging technique uses the artifactual signal changes caused by blood flow to depict the vessel lumen, contrast is not required. Because TOF MRA is flow dependent, absence of signal does not necessarily translate to absence of flow. Rather, blood flow may instead be sluggish and below the critical value.

Flow independent Flow-independent methods for MRA do not rely on contrast or blood flow to generate images. Instead, these images are based on the differences of T1, T2, and chemical shift of the different tissues of the voxel (basic unit of MRI reconstruction that represents a pixel in the display).[11] One of the main advantages of this kind of technique is that the regions of slow flow (ie, stenotic vessel) are imaged more easily as well as avoiding a contrast load and its potential effects on the kidneys.

2-D and 3-D acquisitions 2-D and 3-D MRA imaging exist. 2-D images are obtained and presented in slices from top to bottom. Using sophisticated calculations, 2-D images can be manipulated to become 3-D images. Using this technique, cross-sections from the 2-D images at arbitrary view angles from different slices are used. Although this enhances the 2-D information obtained, this approach results in lower-quality images. Actual 3-D images can be obtained initially, which can be used both in cross-sectional images as well as to display complex vessel geometries where blood is flowing in all spatial directions but requires more spatial encoding and is not available in all centers.[16]

Computerized Tomography/MRI Venogram: Brain/Neck

CT venogram and magnetic resonance venogram (MRV) technology assists with the identification of cerebral venous occlusion. These technologies use computer-assisted generation of images, which result from the difference in signal between flowing blood next to stationary tissue. On an unenhanced CT, indirect signs of cerebral venous thrombosis include intraparenchymal hemorrhage and/or parenchymal edema. A direct sign is called the delta sign. The delta sign occurs when there is hyperdensity in the sagittal sinus on a noncontrast CT image. The reverse finding is noted on a contrast CT when a flow void or hypodensity is noted in the sagittal sinus. Because these findings are subtle, MRV imaging or conventional angiogram is indicated. MRV imaging is both sensitive and specific enough to provide the best noninvasive method of diagnosis for cerebral venous thrombosis although it is prone to artifact caused by slow flow or methemoglobin. Although IV contrast is helpful, diagnosis can occur without contrast instillation. T2-hyperintense (white) signal abnormality may be observed in the distribution of the draining sinus. Normal variations (such as hypoplasia of a transverse sinus) may simulate venous sinus thrombosis. In this situation, conventional arteriography with contrast may be warranted.[17]

Computerized Tomography/MRI Perfusion

PWI and DWI were developed in the late 1980s with the evolution into helical and spiral multislice technology. With this evolution, translation into clinical utilization has occurred. Intuitively it seemed that blood flow disorders could be studied with perfusion techniques. In animal studies, reproducibility, reliability, and accuracy have been noted to be high quality.[18] Despite the fascination with this technology, controversy and varying levels of scientific scrutiny remain. Specific concerns lie with the translation of results into predicting patient outcome or the use of these results in planning treatment.[18]

Perfusion is defined as a steady state delivery of blood to an element of tissue.[11] PWIs help characterize tissue-level blood flow while providing insight into blood delivery to the brain parenchyma. In concept, this technology evaluates blood flow through brain tissue with dead tissue noted to be without flow and areas of risk noted to have sluggish flow. For example, in a stroke patient, demonstration of normal CBF would indicate revascularization has occurred and no acute intervention is necessary. Neurologic dysfunction is noted to occur if CBF falls below 18 mL/100 g to 20 mL/100 g of tissue per minute with infarction occurring after only a few minutes of flow less than 10 mL/100 g. Levels of 10 mL/100 g to 20 mL/100 g, however, may take minutes to hours before cell death occurs. Using this knowledge as a foundation, the theory is that if this intermediate zone of flow could be identified, interventions to focus on quick restoration or optimization of flow may preserve tissue. Problematic to this concept is that restoration of blood flow to arteries serving infarcted or ischemic arteries has been noted to produce reperfusion injury with resultant mass effect that could translate to herniation and possibly death. Thus, risk-benefit evaluation of increased perfusion techniques, including artery recanalization, remains under study to determine which vessels and size of infarct might have a positive impact on a patient's clinical situation.[19,20]

Pathophysiology/physics

In both CTP and MRP, precontrast and postcontrast images are evaluated for the presence of a mismatch to determine potentially salvageable tissue. To better understand the principles behind this, knowledge of autoregulation is helpful. Vascular autoregulation is the neurobiochemical mechanism that works to maintain cerebral perfusion despite changes in local neuronal metabolic activity. Blood sensitivity to blood pressure, blood carbon dioxide, and pH are involved. Changes in these parameters effect local blood flow (ie, high levels of CO_2 cause vasodilatation). In the event of ischemia, decreased perfusion pressure occurs, which prolongs the MTT in both the ischemic core and the penumbra. Because the ischemia has an impact on the integrity of cells, autoregulation induces vasodilatation of capillaries in an attempt to maintain CBF. As a result, CBV in the penumbral tissue stays the same or is increased but the infarct core loses this autoregulation ability and CBF is diminished.[19] Perfusion imaging is generally used to evaluate vascular presentations; however, ischemia can be seen in nonvascular specific territories that indicate other clinical scenarios may be occurring. Examples of these situations include seizure, subdural hematoma, neoplasm, vasospasm, and venous thrombosis.[20]

Computerized tomography perfusion

CTP imaging relies on the speed of multidetector row scanners to follow the entry and exit of radiographic dye through a section of tissue. Acquisition of data begins 4 to 6 seconds after injection and before the contrast reaches the tissue of interest to get a baseline. Perfusion studies are obtained 70 to 90 seconds after injection. Imaged volume is selected at the level of the basal ganglia, which includes anterior, posterior, and middle cerebral vessels. As the contrast passes through the tissue, signal intensities are noted and translate to several perfusion parameters: CBF, CBV, MTT, and TTP. CBF is the volume of blood moving through the mass tissue. CBV is the total volume of blood in the mass tissue. MTT is the average transit time of blood through the mass tissue and TTP is the time from contrast arrival to peak enhancement of the mass tissue.[21] Mismatched images of CBF and CBV and of MTT and TTP indicate a perfusion deficit with tissue noted at risk (**Table 4**).

Magnetic resonance perfusion

Several techniques for MRP exist. Bolus contrast tracking is the most common and quantifies the amount of contrast that reaches the brain tissue after a fast IV bolus injection. Signal intensity (concentration) versus a time curve that tracks the time of bolus transit is used to calculate the physiologic parameters discussed previously (CBF, CBV, MTT, and TTP). Currently there is no standard as to which parameters should be used but MTT and TTP are used most commonly (**Table 5**).[15] Study of the clinical applicability of mismatched tissue on CTP and MRP is ongoing.

Specific questions regarding what to do with this mismatch that are currently under investigation include whether delayed thrombolysis can be used, whether recannulation therapy would be of benefit, and whether pressure or volume augmentation in these patients could improve outcomes.[15] Although perfusion imaging is not required to determine IV lysis or endovascular treatment selection, valid clinical indications do include the following:

- Excluding stroke mimics (hypoglycemia, seizure, complex migraine headaches, conversion disorders, dementia, and brain tumor)
- Identifying early risk for stroke after a transient ischemic attack (TIA)
- Clarifying/confirming the presence or site of vessel occlusion
- Assessment of cerebral vasospasm
- Determining the need for blood pressure management or augmentation in eloquent brain regions
- Guiding disposition decisions, such as ICU placement or frequency of neurologic checks
- Guiding prognosis discussions by more objectively defining the risk/benefit of treating certain pathology[6]

Cerebral Angiography

As discussed previously, the concept of angiography was born in 1931. After years of experimentation, Moniz described contrast-enhanced arteriography as a means to further highlight brain structures. To access the arteries, he used a cut down technique of the carotid arteries, the site of contrast instillation. Vanity and concerns regarding potentially visible neck scarring prevented rapid acceptance initially. In 1944, however, the concept was revisited by Engeset[1] and arteriography became a universally accepted technique to provide images of neck and cerebral blood vessels to evaluate

Table 4			
Cerebral perfusion changes in infarct and penumbra			
Tissue Impact	**Cerebral Blood Volume[b]**	**Cerebral Blood Flow**	**Mean Transit Time[a]**
Ischemic penumbra	Normal or increased	Decreased	Increased
Infarct	Decreased	Decreased	Increased

[a] Parameter that is most accurate for describing penumbral tissue within first few hours after onset of ischemic event.
[b] Parameter that most accurately describes infarct core.

Table 5
CT perfusion versus magnetic resonance perfusion

	CT Perfusion	Magnetic Resonance Perfusion
Advantages	• Superior quantitative accuracy of hemispheric side-to-side comparison • Wide availability • Lower cost • Lower technologic requirements • Shorter imaging time • Superior for detection of arterial patency • 3-D reconstruction and source images provide images comparable to angiography • Superior in evaluating both intracranial and extracranial circulation • Preferred method for evaluation of thrombolysis because the presence of hemorrhage can be ruled out as well	• Offers whole-brain coverage • Does not involve radiographs so preferable for younger patients to reduce lifelong radiation exposure • Can perform without contrast • Superior for detection of small lacunar infarcts and posterior fossa ischemia • More sensitive for evaluation of microhemorrhage
Disadvantages	• Uses x-ray technology that translates to radiation exposure • Uses iodinated contrast	• Cannot be used with mechanical implants, electronically operated devices, pacemakers • Less availability • Higher cost • Longer time to image acquisition • Patient size limitations

for vascular malformations, aneurysms, arterial or venous occlusions, cessation of cerebral flow for brain death evaluation, tumor vasculature, and vasospasm.

Physics

Patients undergoing angiography are placed on a table within a radiology suite or operating room with radiology capabilities. A catheter is inserted into the femoral artery and threaded through the circulatory system into the carotid artery and then cerebral vessels. Intermittently throughout the procedure, a contrast agent is injected into the vessels to enhance visualization of vessel anatomy. Radiographs are taken in a series first as the contrast spreads from the arterial system and another as the contrast reaches the venous system. Although CTA and MRA technology is rapidly improving and may soon achieve similar imaging results, angiography is currently considered the gold standard for visualization of cerebral vessels.

Advantages

- High-quality images
- Ability to treat pathology at time of identification

Disadvantages

- Requires the presence of specialty trained practitioners to perform
- Expensive and not readily available in all facilities
- Requires a contrast load that may cause renal insult or allergic reactions

- Radiation exposure during image acquisition
- Invasive and thus has inherent potential complications associated with it (ie, vascular injury and thrombus invasion with subsequent emboli)

Clinical applications

Given the variety of imaging options available, it is important to be able to choose the best option for the various clinical situations. Patient-specific comorbidities and situations must always be considered when choosing specific testing, with discussion of these specifics beyond the scope of this article. General clinical scenarios are listed.

Computerized Tomography Imaging

CT is the preferred initial screening technique for patients in the acute setting of suspected trauma, stroke, and altered mental status or neurologic changes (**Fig. 21**). It is also the preferred first-line study for the identification of brain tumors (**Fig. 22**). CT imaging is also recommended for suspected bone trauma or the need for detailed bone evaluation. In trauma patients, the presence or absence of blood is quickly noted. In stroke patients, unenhanced CT can reveal the presence of infarct or intracranial hemorrhage as a screen for potential thrombolytic treatment. In the presence of acute stroke, edematous changes or hypodensities are less likely to be seen versus those that may be seen on an acute MRI; however, loss of gray/white differentiation may be seen. Indirect signs of vessel occlusion or slower flow can include a dense MCA sign. Because the proximal MCA travels in the axial plane, hyperdensity of a thrombosed or slow-flow vessel may be seen (**Fig. 23**).[6] In the setting of altered mental status, CT can be used with and without contrast to evaluate for pathology (stroke/trauma), discussed previously, as well as the presence of tumor or abscess as a source of neurologic changes.

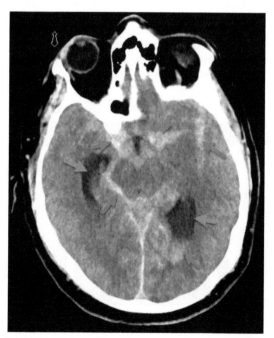

Fig. 21. CT subarachnoid hemorrhage/intraventricular hemorrhage. Blue arrow, intraventricular hemorrhage; green arrows, ventricular CSF; and red arrows, subarachnoid hemorrhage.

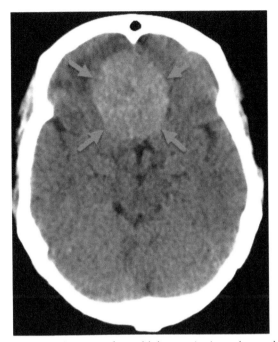

Fig. 22. CT tumor. CT head of anterior frontal lobe meningioma (*arrows*).

CTA expands the role of CT in the acute setting by offering details of major vessels after a bolus of IV contrast. This technology serves to detect proximal large vessel occlusion or injury quickly in stroke and trauma patients. It can also be used to identify underlying vessel abnormalities (ie, arteriovenous malformations or aneurysms), vascular collateral vessels, vasospasm, or tumor vascularization patterns.

In addition to stroke-related mismatches, CTP can be used to exclude stroke mimics (such as Todd paralysis after seizure or metabolic abnormalities). When MRI

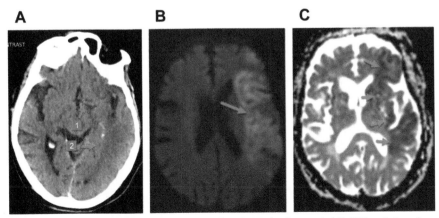

Fig. 23. CT/MRI left middle cerebral artery ischemic stroke (*arrows*). (*A*) CT head: 1 = dense MCA sign; 2 = loss of gray/white matter differential with cerebral edema. (*B*) MRI diffusion sequence of left middle cerebral artery ischemic stroke. (*C*) MRI ADC of left middle cerebral artery ischemic stroke.

DWI is not available, CTP with CBF maps can assist with identifying hypoperfused regions.[6] Additional indications are listed (see **Table 4**).[22]

Primary indications

1. Acute head trauma
2. Suspected acute intracranial hemorrhage
3. Vascular occlusive disease or vasculitis (including use of CTA and/or venography)
4. Aneurysm evaluation
5. Detection or evaluation of calcification
6. Immediate postoperative evaluation after surgical treatment of tumor, intracranial hemorrhage, or hemorrhagic lesions
7. Treated or untreated vascular lesions
8. Suspected shunt malfunctions or shunt revisions
9. Mental status change
10. Increased intracranial pressure
11. Headache
12. Acute neurologic deficits
13. Suspected intracranial infection
14. Suspected hydrocephalus
15. Congenital lesions (such as, but not limited to, craniosynostosis, macrocephaly, and microcephaly)
16. Evaluating psychiatric disorders
17. Brain herniation
18. Suspected mass or tumor

Secondary indications

1. When MRI is unavailable or contraindicated or if the supervising physician deems CT appropriate
2. Diplopia
3. Cranial nerve dysfunction
4. Seizures
5. Apnea
6. Syncope
7. Ataxia
8. Suspicion of neurodegenerative disease
9. Developmental delay
10. Neuroendocrine dysfunction
11. Encephalitis
12. Drug toxicity
13. Cortical dysplasia and migration anomalies or other morphologic brain abnormalities[23–25]

MRI

MRI is rarely done as the initial neuroradiographic evaluation. Generally it follows an initial CT screening. MRI is the preferred method, however, for ischemic stroke (see **Fig. 23**), mass identification (benign/malignant/abscess), and edema evaluation. MRI is also more sensitive for visualization of posterior brain structures. Posterior fossa brain structures are only visualized on several slices of CT imaging due to bone artifact. Therefore, MRI is the study of choice for posterior fossa evaluation (**Fig. 24**). Although CT scan is the initial brain trauma evaluation mode, MRI is best

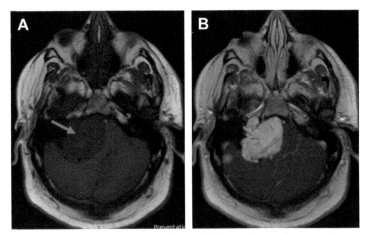

Fig. 24. MRI T1 with/without contrast, right cerebellopontine angle tumor (*arrows*). (*A*) T1 without contrast. (*B*) T1 with contrast.

to identify blood of varying stages and to determine the presence of diffuse axonal injury. MRI is also best for evaluation of neuromuscular diseases and for the evaluation of multiple sclerosis plaques.

Angiography

Angiography is the preferred study for evaluation of aneurysm, arteriovenous malformations, vascular malformations, venous thrombosis, vasculitis, and vasospasm.

There are times when CT, MRI, and angiography imaging are all needed. Each technique excels in different areas but at times the combined techniques optimize a focused patient approach to various care situations. Contrast imaging is suggested if an initial study suggests a tumor or potential infectious cause. Contrast is also suggested in the setting of seizures or in patients with a history of cancer.

SUMMARY

Neurologic imaging has brought intracranial structures from being a dark continent into the light. Through technologic advances, what once took days to obtain can now be completed in a matter of minutes. Single-plane images can now be obtained in multiple visual planes, providing increased information and at times 3-D information on brain pathology or anatomic structures. The wide availability of many of these techniques with varying costs and times for acquisition presents several options when practitioners look to answer questions regarding differential diagnosis. When to use which radiographic technique varies by diagnosis but often requires an overlap of the repertoire to achieve the information desired. Ongoing study and evolution of techniques must be focused toward the optimization, standardization, and clinical validation of how this technology can ultimately have an impact on care of cerebral pathology.

REFERENCES

1. Bull JWD. Section of the history of medicine. Proc R Soc Med 1970;63:637–43.

2. Hickey J, Kanuski JT. Overview of neuroanatomy and neurophysiology. In: Hickey J, editor. The clinical practice of neurological and neurosurgical nursing. 7th edition. Philadelphia: Lippinott Williams & Wilkins; 2014. p. 112–85.
3. Runge VM, Smoker WRK, Valavanis A. Brain. In: Runge VM, Smoker WRK, Valavanis A, editors. Neuroradiology: the essentials with MR and CT. New York: Thieme Medical Publishers, Inc; 2015. p. 1–89.
4. Erkonen WE, Magnotta VA. Radiography, computed tomography, magnetic resonance imaging, and ultrasonography: principles and indications. In: Erkonen WE, Smith WL, editors. Radiology 101: the basics and fundamentals of imaging. 3rd edition. Philadelphia: Wolters Kluwer/Lippincott Williams & Wilkins; 2010. p. 2–15.
5. Blumenfeld H. Introduction to clinical neuroradiology. In: Blumenfeld H, editor. Neuroanatomy through clinical cases. Sutherland (MA): Sinauer Associates, Inc; 2010. p. 85–123.
6. Johnson JM, Lev MH. Acute stroke imaging. In: The stroke book. 2nd edition. Cambridge, United Kingdom: Cambridge University Press; 2013. p. 93–174.
7. Kim YJ, Chang KH, Song IC, et al. Brain abscess and necrotic or cystic brain tumor: discrimination with signal intensity on diffusion-weighted MR imaging. AJR Am J Roentgenol 1998;171:1487–90.
8. Knipe H, Niknejad MT, et al. Apparent diffusion coefficient. Available at: http://radiopaedia.org/articles/apparent-diffusion-coefficient-1. Accessed May 29, 2015.
9. Huisman TAGM. Focus on: diffusion and functional imaging. Diffusion-weighted and diffusion tensor imaging of the brain, made easy. Cancer Imaging 2010; 10:S163–71.
10. Perfusion primer. Available at: http://neuroangio.org/neuroangio-topics/perfusion-primer/. Accessed May 29, 2015.
11. The free dictionary by farlex. Available at: http://medical-dictionary.thefreedictionary.com/. Accessed June 28, 2015.
12. Answers staff. Medical marvels: Cat scan history. Available at: http://invent.answers.com/medical/medical-marvels-cat-scan-history. Accessed July 15, 2015.
13. Jones J. MRI (introduction). Available at: http://radiopaedia.org/articles/mri-introduction. Accessed July 15, 2015.
14. Enterline DS. CT angiography of the neck and brain. In: Kalra MK, Saini S, Rubin GD, editors. MDCT from protocols to practice. Verlag (Italy): Springer; 2008. p. 279–94.
15. Selim MH. Magnetic resonance imaging in acute stroke. In: The stroke book. 2nd edition. Cambridge, United Kingdom: Cambridge University Press; 2013. p. 124–38.
16. Magnetic resonance angiography. Available at: https://en.wikipedia.org/wiki/Magnetic_resonance_angiography. Accessed August 4, 2015.
17. Available at: emedicine.medscape.com/article/338750-overview.
18. Latchaw RE, Yonas H, Hunter GJ, et al. Guidelines and recommendations for perfusion imaging in cerebral ischemia: a scientific statement for healthcare professionals by the writing group on perfusion imaging, from the council on cardiovascular radiology of the American Heart Association. Stroke 2003;34: 1084–104.
19. Leiva-Salinas C, Provenzale JM, Wintermark M. Responses to the 10 most frequently asked questions about perfusion CT. AJR Am J Roentgenol 2011; 196:53–60.
20. D'Esterre CD, Fainardi E, Aviv RI, et al. Improving acute stroke management with computed tomography perfusion: a review of imaging basics and applications. Transl Stroke Res 2012;3:205–20.

21. Major NM. Neuroimaging. In: Major NM, editor. A practical approach to radiology. Philadelphia: Saunder Elsevier; 2006. p. 133–53.
22. Essig M, Shiroishi MS, Nguyen TB, et al. Perfusion MRI: the five most frequently asked technical questions. AJR Am J Roentgenol 2013;200:24–34.
23. National guideline clearinghouse. ACR-ASNR practice guideline for the performance of computed tomography (CT) of the brain. Available at: http://www.guideline.gov/content.aspx?id=32518. Accessed August 14, 2015.
24. Provenzale JM. Imaging of traumatic brain injury: a review of the recent medical literature. AJR Am J Roentgenol 2010;194:16–9.
25. Booya F, Roemro J. Efficient approach to intracerebral hemorrhage: what every radiologist should know: a simple algorithm. AJR Am J Roentgenol 2011; 196(5). http://dx.doi.org/10.2214/ajr.196.5_supplement.a226?src=recsys.

Management of Refractory Intracranial Pressure

Jennifer D. Robinson, MS, APRN, RN, CNRN

KEYWORDS

- Intracranial pressure • Monitoring • Nursing • Neurocritical care

KEY POINTS

- Refractory intracranial pressure (ICP) is a medical emergency and requires immediate attention from medical and nursing staff.
- ICP management is based on a 3-tier approach: medical therapy, metabolic suppression, and surgery.
- Expert nursing assessment and intervention are of vital importance to optimize clinical outcomes in patients with refractory ICP.

OVERVIEW

Intracranial pressure (ICP) is defined as greater than 20 mm Hg sustained for more than 5 minutes in a nonstimulated patient.[1] Common diagnoses that result in elevated ICP include traumatic brain injury, intracranial hemorrhage, and ischemia.[2] Intracranial hypertension is potentially life threatening if not immediately corrected. Refractory intracranial hypertension leads to a reduction of cerebral perfusion.[3] In the most severe cases, refractory intracranial hypertension will result in a complete lack of cerebral perfusion and cause brain death.[3] Utmost importance must be given to effective treatment to correct the abnormality to best improve both patient morbidity and mortality. Bedside nurses should be aware of patients who could potentially develop elevated ICPs and may benefit from an ICP monitor (**Box 1**).[2]

Nurses should be on alert for signs and symptoms of pending intracranial hypertension. Signs and symptoms can be variable and based on the location of the intracranial abnormality; however, the most common symptom is worsening of mental status.[4] Patients often become increasingly more somnolent with elevated ICPs and will progress to coma. Patients should have a baseline head computed tomographic (CT) scan and a repeat head CT scan within 24 hours, and new imaging should be obtained if the patient has an examination change.[5] Patients with brain damage have a 2-fold insult: the initial or primary injury that is irreversible and secondary injury that occurs hours to days after the primary injury.[6] The focus of medical and nursing intervention for these

Neuroscience, Yale New Haven Hospital, 360 State Street #1207, New Haven, CT 06510, USA
E-mail address: jennifer.robinson@yale.edu

Crit Care Nurs Clin N Am 28 (2016) 67–75
http://dx.doi.org/10.1016/j.cnc.2015.09.004
0899-5885/16/$ – see front matter © 2016 Elsevier Inc. All rights reserved.

Box 1
Common diagnosis resulting in elevated intracranial pressure

Diagnosis

Traumatic brain injury

Large territory ischemic stroke

Intraparenchymal hemorrhage

Subarachnoid hemorrhage

Subdural hematoma

Epidural hematoma

Encephalopathy causing cerebral edema

---

patients is on prevention or minimizing the secondary injury. A great reference for nurses is the Brain Trauma Foundation guidelines that were most recently revised in 2007. Hospitals that strictly adhere to these evidence-based guidelines have shown improved mortality and outcomes.[7]

An ICP monitor is commonly placed in patients with a poor neurologic examination and for those at risk for developing elevated ICPs.[8] The particular type of monitor may vary from institution to institution, and the most frequently used devices will be reviewed in this article. An external ventricular drain (EVD) sits in a lateral ventricle and both drains cerebrospinal fluid (CSF) and monitors ICP. An EVD is usually placed in the nondominant hemisphere to minimize potential damage caused in the event of a catheter-induced hemorrhage.[2] An intraparenchymal monitor resides in brain tissue, continuously measures ICP, and can be sophisticated enough to measure brain temperature, brain tissue oxygenation, and other variables but does not drain CSF. **Table 1** further illustrates the differences between an EVD and an intraparenchymal monitor.

The brain is composed of 3 components: brain, blood, and CSF. Reduction of 1 of the 3 is necessary to reduce ICP and forms the basis of the Monro-Kellie hypothesis.[3] CSF drainage via an EVD is the least invasive way to reduce overall brain volume; consequently, an EVD is the most commonly placed device. Consideration is also given to the cerebral perfusion pressure (CPP). CPP is calculated by subtracting ICP from the mean arterial pressure (MAP): $CPP = MAP - ICP$. Maintaining a CPP ideally 60 to 80 mm Hg but not lower than 50 mm Hg is also a strategy used by some institutions.[2]

Table 1
Differences between an external ventricular drain and an intraparenchymal monitor

Device Type	Location	CSF Drainage	Challenges	Continuous ICP Monitoring
EVD	Lateral ventricle ideally in nondominant hemisphere	Yes	Hard to place in patients with small ventricles	No; either drains or monitors; must turn stop cock for accurate reading
ICP monitor	Intraparenchymal (1 cm depth) in same hemisphere as most damaged area	No	No ability to drain CSF	Yes; plus capability to monitor brain tissue oxygen and temperature

CPP and ICP are an indirect measure of cerebral blood flow (CBF).[6] CBF provides the essential nutrients like glucose and oxygen for metabolic demands.[6] Leading experts in neurocritical care raise important discussion points regarding determining an individual patient's point on the cerebral autoregulation curve. For patients with brain injury, their ability to autoregulate their CBF is impaired. See **Fig. 1** for comparison.

In a normal brain, changes in volume are well tolerated, and pressure does not increase until a large volume, approximately 150 mL, is added.[6] In patients with severe brain injury, a small amount of additional volume leads to dramatic increase in ICP; these are the patients who develop refractory intracranial hypertension.

MANAGEMENT

Although the focus of this article is on in-hospital management, recognition should be given to prehospital treatment of the severely brain injured. Care begins in the field with fluid resuscitation to eliminate hypotension and securing of the airway. Avoiding hypoxia and hypotension is vital because both are associated with worse outcomes.[6]

On arrival to the emergency department, clinicians act accordingly to maintain a Pao_2 greater than 60 mm Hg and systolic blood pressure greater than 90 mm Hg.[6] Vital signs are monitored closely, and serial neurologic examinations and neurology and neurosurgery consults are performed rapidly to identify if the patient needs immediate neurosurgical intervention.[6] Basic laboratory tests, including glucose, toxicology screens, complete blood counts, coagulation profile, and arterial blood gas, are obtained. Any coagulopathy should be immediately reversed. A noncontrast head CT is needed as quickly as possible. If the patient is deemed not an immediate surgical candidate, admission to a neuroscience intensive care unit (ICU) is appropriate. For patients with a lesion that requires immediate surgical intervention to prevent herniation, going directly from the emergency department to the operating room is common because time is precious.

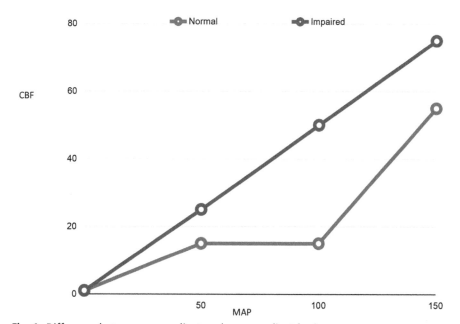

Fig. 1. Difference between a compliant and noncompliant brain.

ICU management continues to focus on the prevention of hypotension and hypoxia. Even a single episode of systolic blood pressure less than 90 is associated with increased mortality.[7,8] Similarly, periods of hypoxia, either O_2 saturation less than 90% or a Pao_2 less than 60 mm Hg, are predictive of both increased morbidity and increased mortality.[6]

ICP management is not consistent worldwide or even within individual ICUs.[9] Although evidence is lacking on the ideal ICP maximum to improve patient outcome, ICP less than 20 mm Hg is standard.[6] Some hospitals use an ICP goal; others use a CPP goal, and some use both. The most frequent variables include EVD versus intraparenchymal device, height of drain, target ICP, and how to lower ICP.[9] Nurses are granted much responsibility for how to correctly place the height of the drain, ICP monitoring, and if necessary, lowering the ICP. Clinicians often enter orders stating "notify team for sustained ICP greater than 20 mm Hg" or "ICP goal less than 20 mm Hg." However, there is variability on how to accomplish this task. A common scenario when an ICU nurse encounters an elevated ICP reading is to first check the patient to ensure an accurate reading. An elevated reading in an alert and talking patient may not be alarming and could indicate an error in the monitor. If the clinical examination correlates with the monitor, the nurse notifies the medical team of the reading. Often, the head of the bed is checked to make sure it is at 30°; the head is placed in a neutral position; CSF is drained if able from an EVD; sedation or analgesics are bolused or increased; and osmotic agents are prepared to be hung. These interventions occur quickly, simultaneously, and often before the medical team arrives.[10]

INTERVENTIONS

Management of elevated ICPs is based on a 3-tier approach[2] (**Table 2**). Optimizing medical therapy forms the basis of the first tier. Patients with either elevated ICP or concern for immediate deterioration should have a secure airway. For patients not intubated, the bedside nursing can plan for both intubation and ventilator settings to ensure eucapnia and adequate oxygen to avoid hypoxia.[3] End-tidal carbon dioxide monitors can be helpful when correlated to the PCO_2 obtained during an arterial blood gas test. Hypotension should be avoided to help prevent secondary brain injury. Anticipating the need for fluid resuscitation, placement of arterial lines and central lines, and vasopressor administration are helpful for this patient population. Blood pressure goals of a systolic pressure greater than 90 mm Hg and MAP greater than 70 mm Hg are best.[2] Additional nursing-driven initiatives for the brain-injured critically ill patients include glucose control to avoid both hypoglycemia and hyperglycemia.[3] The institution should be consulted for exact blood glucose levels, but serum glucose targets of 80 to 180 mg/dL are common.[3] Clinicians should have a low threshold to start a continuous infusion of insulin to achieve this goal. Many hospitals have nursing-driven protocols for glucose control. Isotonic fluids, preferably normal saline,

Table 2		
Management of elevated intracranial pressure		
Tier	Type	Specifics
Tier 1	Medical	Mannitol & hypertonic saline
Tier 2	Metabolic suppression	Hypothermia & barbiturate coma
Tier 3	Surgery	Hemicraniectomy or bifrontal craniectomy
Emergency	Active herniation	Hyperventilation, CSF drainage, or hemicraniectomy

should be infused to prevent increased cerebral edema with use of hypotonic solutions. Acutely brain-injured patients should never have hypotonic saline running.[10]

Additional measures to maintain normothermia and adequate sedation again are classified in the nursing realm.[11] See subsequent text for more on fever control. Sedation and analgesia are ordered by the medical team and administered by the bedside nurse. The nurse decides the amount of both medications and balances obtaining a quality neurologic examination with oversedation or undersedation.[12] Sedation with a short half-life is preferable so providers can obtain frequent neurologic examinations. Propofol is the drug of choice for patients who need frequent neurologic checks.[2]

Other noninvasive strategies for ICP reduction are maintaining the head of the bed elevated to 30°, maintaining a neutral head position, and ensuring the cervical collar is not too tight to decrease jugular venous return.[3] Two fingers should be able to fit inside a cervical collar. The 2 medicines used to reduce refractory ICP are mannitol 20% and hypertonic saline.[6] Both are effective and used frequently in patients with elevated ICPs. Mannitol is dosed at 1 g/kg and infused as quickly as possible. Mannitol loses effectiveness with doses too close together in frequency or with prolonged administration. At present, no blood tests exist to determine the level of accumulated mannitol in the bloodstream. As a result, facilities commonly derive a mannitol level to determine the safety of redosing mannitol. Mannitol crystalizes in the renal tubules so frequent administration and use in renal-compromised patients should be avoided. The best practice to determine if mannitol is safe to redose is to calculate an osmolar gap. Osmolar gap can be calculated by more than one formula, but a common option is[2]:

Calculated osmolality: 1.86(Na + K) + (glucose/18) + (BUN [blood urea nitrogen]/2.8) + 10

Osmolar gap = measured osmolality − calculated osmolality

Orders to administer mannitol will usually have hold parameters for gap greater than 10, Osm greater than 320, or Na greater than 160. The local institution should be consulted for specific practice.

Nurses are also asked to send laboratory tests frequently in order to calculate the osmolar gap. An astute nurse knows the timing of these laboratory tests draws is important because they affect the ability of the next given dose of mannitol. Best practice is to draw the samples as close as possible to the next dose.

Hypertonic saline comes in various concentrations; 1.5%, 3%, and 23.4% are the 3 most common. The lower concentrations are given in a continuous infusion, whereas the highly concentrated formula is given as a bolus. Both hypertonic saline and mannitol reduce ICP. Saline (23.4%) is given as a 30-mL bolus over 10 minutes. They can be used to complement each other. For patients refractory to ICPs, nurses can anticipate administering these medications every few hours.[2] In addition, routine laboratory tests, such as a basic metabolic panel and osmolality, are needed to know if the next dose of mannitol is safe to give. For patients on hypertonic saline therapy only, frequent sodium draws are required to ensure the sodium does not fluctuate dramatically or increase beyond the goal sodium determined by the medical team.

For patients with refractory ICPs despite the first tier of medical management, one moves rapidly to the second tier: metabolic suppression.[2] Two options exist to suppress cerebral metabolic demand: barbiturate administration or hypothermia. Pentobarbital is the most commonly used barbiturate for ICP crisis. A loading dose of 5 to 10 mg/kg is given and may be repeated. Nurses should monitor closely for hypotension given the loading dose because many patients have difficulty tolerating a bolus of pentobarbital. Many patients require both additional fluid and vasopressor support while on pentobarbital. A continuous infusion may be started if the bolus dose has the desired effect of ICP reduction. Continuous electroencephalogram (EEG) is necessary while administering pentobarbital to prevent overdosing.[13] Bedside nurses titrate pentobarbital to burst suppression on EEG (1–2 bursts per minute). The infusion may need to be discontinued if severe hypotension is noted or not responsive to fluid or vasopressors. Remember a reduction in CPP is another indication to stop pentobarbital. Also, the half-life of pentobarbital is quite long, 53 to 118 hours, so careful administration is recommended because the effects linger.[14]

Hypothermia of 32°C to 34°C also reduces ICP and is usually maintained for 24 to 72 hours.[6] Rewarming occurs slowly over 12 to 24 hours. Nurses place an indwelling urinary catheter with a temperature probe for continuous monitoring of the patient's temperature. Hypothermia can also cause hypotension but is generally tolerated better than pentobarbital. Other potential problems to watch closely for include shivering, sepsis, and electrolyte abnormalities.[10] Induction of hypothermia should be as fast as possible and enhanced with administration of boluses of cold saline. As a warning, sepsis can be harder to detect during metabolic suppression. Patient temperature will remain constant, but the astute nurse will detect water temperature of the cooling device that is persistently cold. Cultures should be obtained routinely and with any suspicion of infection. Neurocritical care nurses know that shivering is counterproductive to hypothermia and must be avoided. Shivering can cause hyperthermia and a hypercatabolic state, both of which are the exact opposite of the goals of hypothermia therapy. Nurses can apply a warming blanket for surface counterwarming, can increase sedation, or add pharmacologic agents such as meperidine and buspirone to decrease shivering.[10]

The third and final tier for refractory ICPs is surgical decompression.[2] Hemicraniectomy when performed should offer a large craniotomy and adequate durotomy to prevent herniation. Outcomes from surgical decompression are correlated to the timing of the surgery and the severity of the patient's injury. Early and ongoing conversations with neurosurgery are vital to establish a plan for each patient on the threshold of going to the operating room for decompression. If the patient is a surgical candidate, undergoing surgery before herniation is of utmost importance. Herniation occurs when increased pressure displaces brain tissue to another compartment. Family understanding and guidance of the best course of action cannot be emphasized enough because a hemicraniectomy may ensure patient survival but does not necessarily improve functional outcome.[15,16]

Management of refractory ICP must also include the practice of hyperventilation. Hyperventilation has historically been used as a means of decreasing ICP because hyperventilation causes vasoconstriction, reduces blood flow, and is thought to temporarily decrease ICP. This measure should only be used in an emergency and as a means to taking the patient to an intervention: surgery.[6] If hyperventilation is used as a primary management strategy, the patient will develop rebound cerebral edema, and refractory ICPs will be worse. Again, it is only helpful when managing ICP crisis when en route to the operating room.[2]

Nurses working with patients at risk for refractory ICPs need to be able to recognize signs of herniation. All measures should be taken to avoid herniation because herniation is associated with worsening morbidity and increased mortality. Clinical signs of pupillary asymmetry, nonreactive pupils, decerebrate or decorticate posturing, hypertension with bradycardia, and respiratory arrest should be immediately reported.[2,6]

Nursing Management During Period of Normal Intracranial Pressures

Although the theme of this article is refractory ICP management, brief discussion on nursing tasks: oral care, repositioning, endotracheal suctioning, and chest physiotherapy, should also be discussed. During ICP crisis, best practice is to avoid these activities as to limit any additional ICP increase; however, these tasks can be safely performed in times of normal ICPs. As for routine oral care, ICPs at worst have a minimal 1 to 2 mm Hg increase during oral care and 2 to 3 mm Hg increase after oral care.[17]

Endotracheal suctioning is important for ventilated patients to clear secretions and prevent hypoxia. Recent studies have not shown any association with elevation of ICP. ICP can increase with coughing, tracheal irritation, or hypoxia.[17] Patients should be hyperoxygenated before suctioning to prevent hypoxia. Suctioning is best with 1 or 2 passes at most and completed within several seconds.[17]

Patients not in ICP crisis can be safely repositioned every 2 hours and undergo chest physiotherapy (CPT). The goal of frequent repositioning and CPT is to prevent ICU complications such as skin breakdown and alveolar collapse.[17] Whether CPT is done manually or patients are placed on percussion and vibration bed modules, it can be done safely according to a recent multicenter observational study.[17]

For all 3 tasks: CPT, endotracheal suctioning, and oral care, the nurse is in charge of the specifics of when and how to perform them. Much is left to the discretion of the nurse as to how to prevent common ICU complications, yet much of this practice is variable.[9] Highly trained nurses know best how to safely care for their patients and when to avoid routine care in the critically ill.

HYPERTHERMIA

Refractory ICP and nursing management would not be complete without a review of the importance of maintaining normothermia. Fever is usually first detected by a nurse, and fever control is a routine part of the neuroscience ICU nurse. It is well known that fever and outcome are inversely related, meaning the presence of fever translates to a worse outcome. In addition, hyperthermia is associated with increased length of stay, higher mortality, and large infarct sizes.[18,19] Nurses are key in the decision-making as to the timing of giving an intervention, what kind of intervention is necessary, from antipyretics to tepid bathing to cooling devices.[18] A high incidence of patients with traumatic brain injury, ischemic stroke, and hemorrhagic stroke develops fever.[19–21] Although institutions may differ on the definition of a fever, from 37.2°C to more than 39°C, maintaining normothermia of 37°C is key.[19] Nurses are positioned to combat fever by any of the following management strategies: antipyretic administration, reduction of temperature in the room, packing the patient's axilla and groin in ice, tepid bathing, water cooling blankets, noninvasive targeted temperature device, or intravascular cooling devices.[6] The bedside nurse should be empowered by a multidisciplinary team to rapidly use interventions and escalate the type of intervention to ensure normothermia. Hyperthermia protocols can be helpful in guiding novice nurses on the stepwise approach to management of fevers.

Implications for Critical Care Nurses

The need for ICP monitoring can create anxiety for family members. The critical care nurse can alleviate much stress by explaining how the drain works, the importance of continuous monitoring and evaluation, and the ability to treat high ICP. Family members can often become fixated on one number, so an eloquent explanation as to the wide variety of variables that influence each unique patient situation is more helpful than reacting to one single reading.

Critical care nurses with a patient requiring an ICP monitor should be readily available to administer osmotic therapy, travel for an emergent imaging study, start or increase sedation or analgesics, and troubleshoot the ICP monitor. Planning for a potentially unpredictable day is recommended.

SUMMARY

Refractory intracranial hypertension is a medical emergency. Patient survival is dependent on the immediate and effective coordinated care of a multidisciplinary team. Neurocritical care nurses are on the frontlines of combating this devastating problem and often the first medical team member to identify a problem.[22] Instilling best practice of frequent neurologic examination, monitoring ICP, and strategizing to reduce refractory intracranial hypertension form the basis of a foundation to ensure neurocritical care patients receive the best care and the best chance of a good functional recovery.

REFERENCES

1. Tang A, Pandit V, Fennell V, et al. Intracranial pressure monitor in patients with traumatic brain injury. J Surg Res 2015;194:565–70.
2. Latorre JG, Greer DM. Management of acute intracranial hypertension. Neurology 2009;15:193–207.
3. American Association of Neuroscience Nurses. Nursing management of adults with severe traumatic brain injury. Glenview (IL): AANN Clinical Practice Guideline Series; 2008. p. 1–20.
4. Mayer SA, Chong JY. Critical care management of increased intracranial pressure. J Intensive Care Med 2002;17:55–67.
5. Lobato RD, Alen JF, Perez-Nunez A, et al. Value of serial CT scanning and intracranial pressure monitoring for detecting new intracranial mass effect in severe head injury. Neurocirugia 2005;16:217–34.
6. Neurocritical Care Society. The practice of neurocritical care (Kindle locations 3375-3378). Kindle edition. Minneapolis (MN): Neurocritical Care Society; 2015.
7. Chestnut RM, Marshall LF, Klauber RM, et al. The role of secondary brain injury in determining outcome from severe head injury. J Trauma 1993;34:216–22.
8. Marmarou A, Anderson RL, Ward JD, et al. Impact of ICP instability and hypotension on outcome in patients with severe head trauma. J Neurosurg 1991;75:159–66.
9. Olson DM, Lewis LS, Bader MK, et al. Significant practice pattern variations associated with intracranial pressure monitoring. J Neurosci Nurs 2013;45(4):186–93.
10. Brain Trauma Foundation, American Association of Neurological Surgeons, Congress of Neurological Surgeons, et al. Guidelines for the management of severe traumatic brain injury. Introduction. J Neurotrauma 2007;24(Suppl 1):S1–106.
11. McGrane S, Pandharipande PP. Sedation in the intensive care unit. Minerva Anestesiol 2012;78:369–80.
12. Brook AD, Ahrens TS, Schaiff R, et al. Effect of a nursing-implemented sedation protocol on the duration of mechanical ventilation. Crit Care Med 1999;27:2609–15.
13. Bader MK, Arbour R, Palmer S. Refractory intracranial pressure in severe traumatic brain injury: barbiturate coma and bispectral index monitoring. AACN Clin Issues 2005;16(4):526–41.
14. Nelson E, Powell JR, Conrad K, et al. Phenobarbital pharmacokinetics and bioavailability in adults. J Clin Pharmacol 1982;22(2–3):141–8.

15. Cooper DJ, Rosenfeld JV, Murray L, et al. Decompressive craniectomy in diffuse traumatic brain injury. N Engl J Med 2011;364:1493.

16. Cooper DJ, Rosenfeld JV, Murray L, et al. Early decompressive craniectomy for patients with severe traumatic brain injury and refractory intracranial hypertension—a pilot randomized trial. J Crit Care 2008;23(3):387–93.

17. McNett MM, Olson DM. Evidence to guide nursing interventions for critically ill neurologically impaired patients with ICP monitoring. J Neurosci Nurs 2013; 45(3):120–3.

18. Thompson HJ, Kirkness CJ, Mitcell PH. Fever management practices of neuroscience nurses, part II: nurse, patient, and barriers. J Neurosci Nurs 2007;39(4): 196–201.

19. Thomspson HJ, Kirkness CJ, Mitchell PH, et al. Fever management practices of neuroscience nurses: national and regional perspectives. J Neurosci Nurs 2007; 39(3):151–62.

20. McIlvoy LH. The effect of hypothermia and hyperthermia on acute brain injury. AACN Clin Issues 2005;16:488–500.

21. Kilpatrick MM, Lowery DW, Firlik AD, et al. Hyperthermia in the neurosurgical intensive care unit. Neurosurgery 2000;47:850–6.

22. McNett MM, Gianakis A. Nursing interventions for critically ill traumatic brain injury patients. J Neurosci Nurs 2010;42(2):71–7.

Invasive Neuromonitoring

Carey Heck, PhD, CRNP, ACNP-BC, CCRN, CNRN

KEYWORDS

- Invasive neuromonitoring • Intraparenchymal monitor • External ventricular device
- Multimodal monitoring • Traumatic brain injury

KEY POINTS

- A variety of invasive neuromonitoring devices exist to monitor intracranial pressure (ICP). Device selection is dictated by patient presentation, desired device function, practitioner preference, and institutional policies and is ideally supported by current research.
- The use of invasive neuromonitoring in an effort to improve patient outcomes through prevention of secondary ischemia due to increased ICP is considered the standard of care in neurocritical care management in most developed countries throughout the world.
- The steadfast reliance on ICP monitoring as beneficial in the management of neuroscience patients, despite a paucity of controlled clinical trials supporting such management, is not without controversy in the literature.

INTRODUCTION

Critical care management of neurologic injury has historically focused on prevention of secondary ischemic injury through aggressive management of intracranial pressure (ICP) and maintenance of adequate cerebral perfusion pressure (CPP).[1–3] The concept of ICP was first introduced in 1783 by the Scottish physician, Dr Monro, who described the skull as a rigid box with a fixed volume that was composed of blood, brain tissue, and cerebral spinal fluid (CSF). In 1824, the Scottish surgeon, Dr Kellie, further expanded on this hypothesis by noting that an increase in the volume of one component resulted in a decrease in the volume of the other components. The work by these early physicians is now well known as the Monro-Kellie hypothesis and has significant implications when discussing and managing ICP and invasive neuromonitoring.[4–6] Invasive neuromonitoring in an effort to prevent poor patient outcomes secondary to increased ICP has been the mainstay of neurocritical management for centuries, particularly in the management of patients with traumatic brain injured and subarachnoid hemorrhage (SAH).[1,3,4,6–8]

Despite the unwavering reliance on ICP monitoring, it is essential to observe that significant controversy exists in the literature surrounding this technology.[9–11] Controversy

The author has nothing to disclose.
College of Nursing, Thomas Jefferson University, 901 Walnut Street, Suite 815, Philadelphia, PA 19107, USA
E-mail address: carey.heck@jefferson.edu

Crit Care Nurs Clin N Am 28 (2016) 77–86
http://dx.doi.org/10.1016/j.cnc.2015.10.001
0899-5885/16/$ – see front matter © 2016 Elsevier Inc. All rights reserved.

exists concerning the choice and placement of devices.[12,13] The literature notes controversy surrounding the use of single-device ICP monitoring versus multimodality monitoring.[3,9,14,15] Finally, as a result of the Benchmark Evidence from South American Trials: Treatment of Intracranial Pressure (BEST TRIP) trial,[16] substantial debate has been generated concerning the ultimate benefit of ICP monitoring.[7,8,10,16–18]

RATIONALE FOR INVASIVE NEUROMONITORING

The overarching goal of neurocritical care management is to prevent secondary brain ischemia.[1,5,12,19] Increased ICP has repeatedly been demonstrated to compromise cerebral blood flow leading to cerebral hypoxia and ischemia.[11,19] The negative consequences of increased ICP include increased mortality and morbidity.[1,7,20,21] Conversely, aggressive management and control of ICP have been demonstrated to result in improved neurologic outcomes in patients with traumatic brain injury (TBI).[1,20,21]

Goals of management are generally accepted as maintenance of ICP 20 mm Hg or greater with some practitioners reserving treatment threshold at ICP 25 mm Hg or greater. CPP value goals are generally accepted to be maintained 60 to 70 mm Hg.[1,4,8,22–24] Ultimately, the ICP and CPP reference ranges should be individualized for each patient, taking into consideration underlying abnormality and goals of treatment.[4,22,25,26]

Monitoring of ICP[1,22,24,25]:

- Allows for the rapid recognition of elevated ICP
- Ensures maintenance of optimal CPP
- Assesses the efficacy of therapeutic measures
- Evaluates the evolution of brain injury

INDICATIONS FOR INVASIVE NEUROMONITORING

A variety of disease processes and neurologic conditions warrant the use of invasive neuromonitoring.[4,12,22–26] However, 2 specific populations of neuroscience patients historically have used more frequent invasive neuromonitoring due to their neuropathology and have subsequently dominated research and case study literature.[1,12,27–30] These specific patient populations include patients with severe TBI and patients with SAH as a result of cerebral aneurysmal rupture.

Much of the extant literature on ICP monitoring is focused on the patient with severe traumatic brain injury. The propensity of literature on this specific population, along with the adoption of international guidelines and standardized protocols, has resulted in the acceptance of ICP monitoring as the standard of care for patients with severe TBI at most large trauma centers in developed countries.[1,2,8,29] Use of EVDs for temporary or permanent CSF diversion is recommended in symptomatic patients with chronic hydrocephalus following SAH.[27] Recommendations for ICP monitoring are also noted in evidence-based guidelines for intracerebral hemorrhage.[27,28]

The most common indications include use in patients with[1,7,22–25,27]

- TBI
- SAH
- Intracerebral hemorrhage
- Obstructive hydrocephalus

Other indications include patients with

- Cerebral infections
- Congenital abnormalities

- Mass lesions
- Hepatic failure

INTRACRANIAL MONITORING OPTIONS

A variety of devices are available to monitor ICP. Device selection is dictated by the patient's presentation and desired device function, practitioner preference, and institutional policies and is ideally driven by current best evidence.[12,13]

ICP monitors are classified based on their ultimate location within the brain (**Fig. 1**) and their function (monitoring of ICP alone or monitoring and therapy). Devices inserted directly into the parenchyma are commonly referred to as intraparenchymal monitors (IPM) in the literature. Other less commonly used, and less reliable, monitors are inserted in the potential spaces of the brain (subdural, epidural) and also have ICP monitoring capabilities only. A catheter inserted into the cerebral ventricle and attached to a transducer system allows for monitoring of ICP as well as continuous or intermittent drainage of CSF.[1,3,4,11] The latter devices are collectively referred to as external ventricular devices (EVDs) in the literature. IPMs and EVDs are used most frequently in the clinical setting and are discussed in greater detail in later discussion.[12,26] **Table 1** notes the different types of ICP monitors available in the clinical setting.

Brain tissue oxygen monitoring in the management of neuroscience patients has been a topic of interest in the neurocritical care literature for decades.[7] Advocates of continuous brain oxygen monitoring argue that changes in brain cerebral oxygenation indicating hypoxia and ischemia occur despite the presence of normal ICP and CPP values.[3,7,15] Brain tissue oxygen monitoring as a more complex option for invasive neuromonitoring technology is also discussed in detail later.

Device Insertion

Measurement of ICP is achieved by insertion of devices into the brain parenchyma or the cerebral ventricles.[6,27] Choice of device is based on whether the ultimate goal of management is ICP monitoring alone (for instance in a patient with TBI) in which case

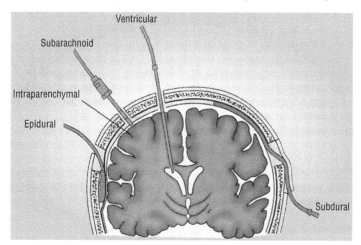

Fig. 1. Placement of invasive neuromonitoring devices. (*Adapted from* Kerr M, Crago EA. Nursing management: acute intracranial problems. In: Lewis SM, Heitkemper MM, Dirksen SR, editors. Medical-surgical nursing: assessment and management of clinical problems, 6th edition. St Louis (MO): CV Mosby; 2004. p. 1918; with permission.)

Table 1
Advantages and disadvantages of intracranial monitors used most frequently in the clinical setting

Type of Monitor	Location	Advantages	Disadvantages

IPM	Parenchyma	Ease of placement
		Less infectious
		  complications
			Cannot be recalibrated
			  once placed
			Fiberoptics are easily
			  damaged
			Cost

EVD	Ventricles	"Gold standard"
		Most reliable and
		  accurate
		Monitoring and therapy
		  via drainage of CSF
		  and blood
		Easily recalibrated in situ
			Technically challenging to
			  insert in certain clinical
			  situations
			Higher risk of
			  complication including
			  infection and
			  hemorrhage
			Obstruction possibility

Subarachnoid screw	—	Ease of placement	—

Subdural	Between dura and
	  subarachnoid
	  space
		Ease of placement
		Low complication risk
			Low rate of complication
			Less reliable
			Poor waveform

Epidural	Between skull and
	  dura
		Ease of placement
		Low complication risk
			Indirect measurement of
			  ICP
			Less reliable
			Poor waveform
			Rarely used

Adapted from Refs.[1,12,24,26,31,32]

an IPM is appropriate. If, however, the management goal is ICP monitoring and drainage of CSF or blood (for instance, in a patient with SAH or in a patient with hydrocephalus), then an EVD would be a more appropriate choice.

A basic understanding of the anatomic landmarks for device insertion as well as the advantages and disadvantages associated with the various devices is necessary and is henceforth described. Insertion of an intracranial monitor is performed in the operating room or at the patient's bedside, although institutional variations may be significant and will be dictated by those policies and procedures. Insertion of any invasive neuromonitoring device carries the risk of infection.[4,12,13,33] The procedure is therefore conducted adhering to strict sterile technique.[4,22] Insertion by a credentialed practitioner may be done using several techniques, although the most common point for ICP monitor insertion is the Kocher point.[13,33]

The Kocher point is located by measuring

- 10.5 to 11 cm back from the nasion
- 2.5 to 3.0 cm lateral to the midline (midpupillary line)

Alternatively, measuring 1 cm anterior of the coronal suture on the midpupillary line is another method to locate Kocher point.[13,33,34]

External Ventricular Devices

Several types of EVD transducers are available in the clinical setting. These transducers include external strain-gauge (ESG), internal strain-gauge, or fiberoptic catheter.[22,24,31] Ventricular catheters connected to an ESG transducer are most commonly used in the clinical setting.[24,31] EVDs can be easily recalibrated, rendering them highly accurate. As noted earlier, EVDs not only allow for measurement of ICP but also have the added benefit of allowing therapeutic interventions through drainage of CSF or blood.[4,11,23,24] For these reasons, EVDs are frequently referred to as the gold standard in ICP monitoring.[4,24]

The literature has noted the advantages of EVDs in the management of both patients with TBI and patients with SAH. As noted earlier, EVDs are beneficial in the management of SAH. The literature has noted that in patients with SAH with hydrocephalus who were clinically compromised, 40% to 80% showed improvement after an EVD was placed, with patients showing evidence of clinical improvement after placement of an EVD.[34–36]

The disadvantages of EVDs are evident when one considers the end location of the device. The device is most frequently placed in the lateral ventricle, and placement can be challenging if the ventricle is compressed due to mass effect or collapsed due to lack of CSF.[12] The literature has also noted an increased risk of hemorrhage and infection when compared with IPM.[12,33] Other investigators, however, have noted no difference in the rate of complication between the 2 device types.[13,37]

Intraparenchymal Monitors

Another method of measuring ICP is through the use of catheters inserted directly into the brain parenchyma. These intraparenchymal devices are used when drainage of CSF is not necessary or when insertion into the ventricle is not possible (in the case of ventricular compression due to cerebral edema, for example). The advantages of IPMs include less technical challenges with device placement and theoretically a lower risk of infection. Disadvantages of IPMs include the inability to recalibrate once the device has been placed and the cost compared with EVDs.

ADVANTAGES AND DISADVANTAGES OF INVASIVE NEUROMONITORING

The decision to use technology is based on consideration of many factors. Patient presentation and the goals of therapy will quite frequently drive the decision for device choice. Technical expertise of the practitioner as well as institutional culture and policies will also be significant considerations. The advantages and disadvantages of the numerous devices available to the practitioner must also be deliberated because these often overlap with the previously mentioned considerations. **Table 1** summarizes the advantages and disadvantages of the most commonly used intracranial monitoring devices.

The decision to place an IPM versus an EVD continues to be debated in the literature. Liu and colleagues[13] in a prospective observational study of patients with TBI found that EVDs may provide an advantage in controlling refractory intracranial hypertension compared with IPMs. However, Kasotakis and colleagues[12] found that IPMs were associated with fewer complications than EVDs in patients with TBI who required ICP monitoring. Kasotakis and colleagues retrospectively reviewed the records of 378 patients with severe TBI admitted to a level I trauma center who required ICP monitoring and found that patients with IPMs were monitored for a shorter amount of time, had a decreased length of stay in the intensive care unit, and had a lower rate of device-related complications compared with patients with EVDs. The investigators noted no difference in device selection and neurologic outcomes.

Brain Tissue Oxygen Monitoring

Monitoring intracranial volume changes alone, which is the only information derived from IPMs and EVDs, may be inadequate for the practitioner tasked with managing critically ill neuroscience patients. It has been demonstrated that ICP monitoring alone misses the dynamic changes in oxygen delivery and consumption that occur before clinical signs are evident in a patient's assessment.[3,14,32] Additional physiologic information available through brain tissue oxygen ($PbtO_2$) monitoring augments data provided by IPMs and EVDs. $PbtO_2$ monitoring as an adjunctive invasive neuromonitoring detects regional cerebral hypoxia via insertion of specialized probes inserted adjacent to ICP monitoring catheters. The placement of the $PbtO_2$ monitor may be in the white matter on either the injured or the uninjured side of the brain. Placement on the uninjured side of the brain allows for measurement of the effectiveness of therapy and may be allowed for early detection of further ischemic damage.[7,32,38]

The literature defines normal $PbtO_2$ between 25 and 35 mm Hg with initiation of treatment generally recommended for $PbtO_2$ less than 20 mm Hg.[15,25] Interventions are directed toward improving oxygenation in an effort to prevent further ischemia or neuronal death.[32] These interventions may include interventions designed to improve hypotension, hypovolemia, or hypoxia.[15] Interventions to decrease cerebral metabolism are also important and include sedation, pain management, maintenance of normothermia, and seizure prophylaxis.[15]

CONTROVERSIES IN INVASIVE NEUROMONITORING
Does the Evidence Support Practice?

As noted earlier, ICP monitoring based on established guidelines is the accepted standard of care in developed countries for the management in patients with TBI, despite a lack of randomized controlled trials.[39] A positive relationship between patient outcomes and compliance with established guidelines has been reported in the literature. Stein and colleagues[20] reported that higher-intensity treatment with the use of ICP monitoring resulted in lower mortality and a more favorable patient outcome compared with less aggressive treatment and monitoring where ICP monitoring was not used. Gerber and colleagues[21] also reported a decline in mortality when adherence to established guidelines with ICP monitoring and CPP thresholds were observed. Although Yuan and colleagues[18] reported ICP monitoring overall was not significantly superior to no ICP monitoring regarding mortality; subgroup analysis of studies published after 2012 indicated an association between decreased mortality and patients with ICP monitors in place. The investigators suggested that standardized management and rigorous adherence to Brain Trauma Foundation (BTF) guidelines may have been responsible for this finding. However, the rate of compliance with BTF guidelines has been reported to be inconsistent and suboptimal, resulting in several researchers to lament the care received by patients with TBI.[9,30,40] Shafi and colleagues[41] noted that "decades after the establishment of evidence-based guidelines the management of patients with severe traumatic brain injury remains suboptimal." Mendelson and colleagues[30] also noted poor adherence to established guidelines and recommended future studies examining reasons for nonadherence.

ICP monitoring is not without inherent risks.[31,33] If failure to follow established guidelines designed to facilitate best outcomes is prevalent in clinical practice, reservations concerning the true benefit of the technology arise. Given that evidence exists that questions the benefit of this technology, discussion must ensue to further explore this concern.

A systematic review conducted by Mendelson and colleagues[30] examined the relationship between ICP monitoring and mortality in patients with severe TBI. The researchers were unable to clearly establish an isolated benefit of ICP monitoring in patients with severe TBI. The clear benefit of ICP monitoring has been questioned in other studies as well.[9,10,18]

Careful deliberation when making decisions regarding placement of intracranial monitoring devices is necessary for all patients, but certain patient populations warrant particular mention. The decision to place an ICP monitor may not be in the best interest of all patients when situational contexts are considered this seems to be true for the elderly patient with TBI. The literature has demonstrated that elderly patients with TBI had an increased hospital mortality and unfavorable discharge placement compared with elderly patients who did not have intracranial monitoring. These poor outcomes were found despite management according to BTF guidelines. Although the literature points to the patient who seems to benefit the least from ICP monitoring, the ideal patient candidate for ICP monitoring remains controversial.[10,18] Yuan and colleagues[18] recommends that further research identify "distinct subgroups" of patients who would most benefit from ICP monitoring.

Benchmark Evidence from South American Trials: Treatment of Intracranial Pressure Trial

The most significant evidence contributing to the controversy surrounding the benefit of intracranial monitoring is the BEST TRIP trial.[16] The BEST TRIP trial was a randomized controlled trial that compared the management strategies of patients with severe TBI in Bolivia and Ecuador. Patients were randomized to receive guidelines-based protocol management that included ICP monitoring with an IPM or protocol management based on imaging and clinical examination. The investigators hypothesized that an ICP monitoring-based protocol in patients with severe TBI would result in reduced mortality and improved outcomes. Secondary hypotheses included an expectation for reduced length of stay in the intensive care unit and fewer complications in the patients randomized to the ICP monitored group.

The unexpected results of the BEST TRIP trial suggested that ICP monitoring was not superior to care based on clinical assessment, and imaging further challenged the rote use of ICP monitoring. Although critics of the study have noted study limitations, the standard of ICP monitoring in the management of all patients with severe TBI is worthy of further discussion.[41–43]

A consensus-based interpretation consisting of international experts in the clinical and research care of TBI patient management was convened to address the considerable controversy that arose as a result of the BEST TRIP trial.[17] Of the 7 statements reflecting the group's consensus and conclusions, a strong call for further research on ICP interpretation and research was evident.

Intracranial Pressure Monitoring Alone Versus Multimodal Monitoring

The concern that ICP monitoring may not confer a benefit has been previously discussed and is the subject of much controversy. Much of the controversy argues that ICP monitoring alone should not be the sole source of information on which therapy is guided but should be incorporated into the arsenal of emerging and promising invasive neuromonitoring devices. In addition to ICP monitoring, devices such as $PbtO_2$, cerebral microdialysis, and electrophysiology monitoring are available tools to optimize patient outcomes.[5,8,19,44] This combination of tools is referred to as multimodal monitoring.

Multimodal monitoring has been described as a dynamic process that uses a variety of tools to simultaneously monitor multiple cerebral physiologic data.[7,45,46] The integration of this data allows the practitioner to discretely and precisely adjust therapy based on individual changes to a patient's brain physiology.[3,14,15] In addition, multimodality monitoring has been noted to confer a survival benefit to patients.[7,19,46] Although the evidence for multimodal monitoring and improved patient outcomes is limited, multimodal monitoring appears to offer promise for invasive neuromonitoring options in the care of critical ill neuroscience patients.[3,14,26]

SUMMARY

The use of invasive neuromonitoring in an effort to prevent poor patient outcomes secondary to increased ICP has been fundamental in neurocritical care management. Monitoring of ICP is achieved via a variety of devices including IPMs and EVDs. Each of these devices comes with its own advantages and disadvantages. The decision regarding optimal device selection for a particular patient scenario is made based on thoughtful consideration of many factors.

Despite the unwavering reliance on ICP monitoring, controversy in the literature exists as to the benefit of this technology. Recent studies have demonstrated that therapy driven by ICP monitoring devices may not confer a clear benefit to patients. Numerous researchers have advocated multimodality monitoring as an alternative to ICP monitoring alone. Future research focusing on this promising avenue of invasive neuromonitoring is warranted. As has been demonstrated, the impact of ICP monitoring in the published literature is variable. To determine the ultimate benefit of intracranial monitoring, either alone or as a component of multimodal monitoring, further research is indeed necessary.

REFERENCES

1. Brain Trauma Foundation, American Association of Neurologic Surgeons, Congress of Neurologic Surgeons, et al. Guidelines for the management of severe traumatic brain injury VI: indications for intracranial pressure monitoring. J Neurotrauma 2007;24(Suppl 1):S37–44.
2. Chestnut R, Videtta W, Vespa P, et al. Intracranial pressure monitoring: fundamental considerations and rationale for monitoring. Neurocrit Care 2014; 21(Suppl 2):S64–84.
3. Chen H, Stiefel M, Oddo M, et al. Detection of cerebral compromise with multimodality monitoring in patients with subarachnoid hemorrhage. Neurosurgery 2011; 69:53–63.
4. Slazinski T, Anderson TA, Cattell A, et al. Care of the patient undergoing intracranial pressure monitoring/external ventricular drainage or lumbar drainage. In: AANN clinical practice guideline series. 2011. Available at: http://www.aann. org/pubs/content/guidelines.html. Accessed August 20, 2015.
5. Olson D, Kofke W, O'Phelan K, et al. Global monitoring in the neurocritical care unit. Neurocrit Care 2015;22:333–47.
6. Di Ieva A, Schmitz E, Cusimano M. Analysis of intracranial pressure: past, present, and future. Neuroscientist 2013;19:592–603.
7. Oddo M, Villa F, Citerio G. Brain multimodality monitoring: an update. Curr Opin Crit Care 2012;18:111–8.
8. Mattei T. Intracranial pressure monitoring in severe traumatic brain injury: who is still bold enough to keep sinning against the level I evidence? World Neurosurg 2013;5/6:602–4.
9. Tang A, Pandit V, Fennell V, et al. Intracranial pressure monitor in patients with traumatic brain injury. J Surg Res 2015;194:565–70.
10. Dang Q, Simon J, Catino J, et al. More fateful than fruitful? Intracranial pressure monitoring in elderly patients with traumatic brain injury is associate with worse outcomes. J Surg Res 2015;198(2):482–8.

11. Garton HJ, Lehmann E. Craniocerebral trauma. In: Doherty GM, editor. Current diagnosis & treatment surgery. 13th edition. New York: McGraw Hill; 2010. p. 814–24.
12. Kasotakis G, Michailidou M, Bramos A, et al. Intraparenchymal vs extracranial ventricular drain intracranial pressure monitors in traumatic brain injury: less is more? J Am Coll Surg 2012;214:950–7.
13. Liu H, Wang W, Chen F, et al. External ventricular drains versus intraparenchymal intracranial pressure monitors in traumatic brain injury: a prospective observational study. World Neurosurg 2015;83:794–800.
14. Le Roux P. Intracranial pressure after the BEST TRIP trial: a call for more monitoring. Curr Opin Crit Care 2014;20:141–7.
15. Cecil S, Chen P, Callaway S, et al. Traumatic brain injury: advanced multimodal neuromonitoring from theory to clinical practice. Crit Care Nurse 2011;31:25–36.
16. Chestnut R, Temkin N, Carney N, et al. A trial of intracranial-pressure monitoring in traumatic brain injury. N Engl J Med 2012;367:2471–81.
17. Chestnut R, Bleck T, Citerio G, et al. A consensus-based interpretation of the BEST TRIP ICP trial. J Neurotrauma 2015. http://dx.doi.org/10.1089/neu.2015.3976.
18. Yuan Q, Xing W, Yirui S, et al. Impact of intracranial pressure monitoring on mortality in patients with traumatic brain injury: a systematic review and meta-analysis. J Neurosurg 2015;122:574–87.
19. Nangunoori R, Maloney-Wilensky E, Stiefel M, et al. Brain tissue oxygen-based therapy and outcome after severe traumatic brain injury: a systematic literature review. Neurocrit Care 2012;17:131–8.
20. Stein SC, Georgoff P, Meghan S, et al. Relationship of aggressive monitoring and treatment to improved outcomes in severe traumatic brain injury. J Neurosurg 2010;112:1105–12.
21. Gerber LM, Chiu YL, Carner N, et al. Marked reduction in mortality in patients with severe traumatic brain injury. J Neurosurg 2013;119:1583–90.
22. Leeper B, Lovasik D. Cerebrospinal drainage systems: external ventricular and lumbar drains. In: Littlejohns LR, Bader MK, editors. AACN-AANN protocols for practice: monitoring technologies in critically ill neuroscience patients. Sudbury (Ontario): Jones and Bartlett; 2009. p. 71–82.
23. March K, Madden L. Intracranial pressure management. In: Littlejohns LR, Bader MK, editors. AACN-AANN protocols for practice: monitoring technologies in critically ill neuroscience patients. Sudbury (Ontario): Jones and Bartlett; 2009. p. 35–69.
24. March K. Technology. In: Littlejohns LR, Bader MK, editors. AANN core curriculum for neuroscience nursing. 5th edition. Glenview (IL): American Association of Neuroscience Nurses; 2010. p. 185–95.
25. Hinkle JL, Heck C. Monitoring for neurologic dysfunction. In: Booker KJ, editor. Critical care nursing: monitoring and treatment for advanced nursing practice. Ames (IA): Wiley Blackwell; 2015. p. 87–103.
26. Kirkman MA, Smith M. Intracranial pressure monitoring, cerebral perfusion pressure estimation, and ICP/CPP-guided therapy: a standard of care or optional extra after brain injury? Br J Anaesth 2014;112:35–46.
27. Hemphill JC, Greenberg SM, Anderson CS, et al. Guidelines for the management of spontaneous intracerebral hemorrhage: a guideline for healthcare professionals form the American Heart Association/American Stroke Association. Stroke 2015;46:2032–60.
28. Bederson JB, Connolly ES, Batjer HH, et al. Guidelines for the management of aneurysmal subarachnoid hemorrhage: a statement for healthcare professionals

from a special writing group of the Stroke Council, American Heart Association. Stroke 2009;40:994–1025.

29. Maas AI, Dearden M, Teasdale GM, et al. EBIC-guidelines for management of severe head injury in adults: European Brain Injury Consortium. Acta Neurochir 1997;139:286–94.

30. Mendelson AA, Gillis C, Henderson WR, et al. Intracranial pressure monitors in traumatic brain injury: a systematic review. Can J Neurol Sci 2012;39:571–6.

31. Bekar A, Dogan S, Abas F, et al. Risk factors and complications of intracranial pressure monitoring with a fiberoptic device. J Clin Neurosci 2009;16:236–40.

32. Vender J, Waller J, Dhandapani K, et al. An evaluation and comparison of intraventricular, intraparenchymal, and fluid-coupled techniques for intracranial pressure monitoring in patients with severe traumatic brain injury. J Clin Monit Comput 2011;25:231–6.

33. Muralidharan R. External ventricular drains: management and complications. Surg Neurol Int 2015;6:S271–4.

34. Greenberg MS. Operations and procedures. In: Handbook of neurosurgery. 7th edition. New York: Thieme; 2010. p. 207–14.

35. Rajshekhar V, Harbaugh RE. Results of routine ventriculostomy with external ventricular drainage for acute hydrocephalus following subarachnoid haemorrhage. Acta Neurochir 1992;115:8–14.

36. Hasan D, Vermeulen M, Wijdicks EF, et al. Management problems in acute hydrocephalus after subarachnoid hemorrhage. Stroke 1989;20:747–53.

37. Milhorat TH. Acute hydrocephalus after aneurysmal subarachnoid hemorrhage. Neurosurgery 1987;20:15–20.

38. Mulvey JM, Dorsch N, Mudaliar Y, et al. Multimodality monitoring in severe traumatic brain injury: the role of brain tissue oxygenation monitoring. Neurocrit Care 2004;1:391–402.

39. Blissitt PA. Brain oxygen monitoring. In: Littlejohns LR, Bader MK, editors. AACN-AANN protocols for practice: monitoring technologies in critically ill neuroscience patients. Sudbury (Ontario): Jones and Bartlett; 2009. p. 103–44.

40. Forsyth RJ, Wolny S, Rodrigues B. Routine intracranial pressure monitoring in acute coma. Cochrane Database Syst Rev 2010;(2):CD002043.

41. Shafi S, Barnes SA, Millar D, et al. Suboptimal compliance with evidence-based guidelines in patients with traumatic brain injuries. J Neurosurg 2014;120:773–7.

42. Hutchinson PJ, Kolias AG, Czosnyka M, et al. Intracranial pressure monitoring in severe traumatic brain injury. BMJ 2013;346:f1000.

43. Albuquerque FC. Intracranial pressure monitoring after blunt head injuries: conflicting opinions. World Neurosurg 2013;79:598.

44. Ghajar J, Carney N. Intracranial-pressure monitoring in traumatic brain injury. N Engl J Med 2013;368:1749.

45. Mahdavi Z, Naregnia P, Thuy-Tien H, et al. Advances in cerebral monitoring for the patient with traumatic brain injury. Crit Care Nurs Clin North Am 2015;27:213–23.

46. Maloney-Wilensky E, Gracias V, Itkin A, et al. Brain tissue oxygen and outcome after severe traumatic brain injury: a systematic review. Crit Care Med 2009;37:2057–63.

Principles of Neuro-anesthesia in Neurosurgery for Intensive Care Unit Nurses

Marian Feil, DNP, CRNA, MSN*, Nicole A. Irick, RN, BSN, CCRN

KEYWORDS

- Neuro-anesthesia • Monitoring • Intraoperative management • Complications
- Positioning

KEY POINTS

- Induction of anesthesia is a critical period of time because of the physiologic effects of direct laryngoscopy and endotracheal intubation, which can cause large increases in blood pressure.
- Motor evoked potentials (MEPs) are used to monitor spinal cord tracts spinal surgery. MEPs monitoring is a prognosticator of a patient's postoperative motor function.
- Intraoperative techniques used to lower an elevated intracranial pressure include hyperventilation, cerebral spinal fluid drainage, administering hyperosmotic drugs, diuretics, corticosteroids, and vasoconstricting anesthetic drugs, such as barbiturates and propofol.
- It is important to prevent and manage hypertension during emergence from anesthesia, as this has been linked to postoperative hematoma formation.
- When transferring a patient from the operating room to the intensive care unit, the clinical handoff ensures care continuity and patient safety, as communication failures can lead to uncertainty in decisions about patient care and result in suboptimal care.

INTRODUCTION

As neurosurgical interventions and procedures are advancing, so is the specialty of neuro-anesthesia. Neuro-anesthesia is different than other anesthetic specialties because both the anesthetist and surgeon are focusing on the same organ during a single surgical case.[1] Throughout the surgery, the main priorities of the neuro-anesthetist are patient safety, patient well-being, surgical field exposure, and patient positioning.[2] For the duration of the surgery, neuro-anesthesia requires continuous provider vigilance and frequent intervention.[2] Although each provider has his or her own respective

Disclosures: None.
Thomas Jefferson University, Philadelphia, PA, USA
* Corresponding author.
E-mail address: Marian.Feil@jefferson.edu

Crit Care Nurs Clin N Am 28 (2016) 87–94
http://dx.doi.org/10.1016/j.cnc.2015.10.004
0899-5885/16/$ – see front matter © 2016 Elsevier Inc. All rights reserved.

roles and responsibilities, cooperation and communication between the anesthetist and neurosurgeon can significantly improve the outcome of the surgery.[2]

Furthermore, other goals of neuro-anesthesia include sustaining an acceptable cerebral perfusion to prevent ischemia while making sure that intracranial pressure (ICP) is not increasing or elevated.[1] Lastly, neurosurgery can be categorized into excision of intracranial mass lesions, decompression procedures, spinal procedures, and aneurysm clippings.

PREOPERATIVE EVALUATION

Every neurosurgical patient should be evaluated for signs and symptoms of elevated ICP, which include nausea/vomiting, headache, changes in vision, altered level of consciousness, irregular breathing patterns, hypertension, or bradycardia. The preoperative evaluation should include a review of pertinent medical and surgical histories, medications, allergies, laboratory tests, preoperative fluid and electrolyte status, and airway assessment. Patients' cardiac status should be thoroughly assessed. If patients are thought to be at risk for a cardiac event, an echocardiogram or a cardiac catheterization may be indicated before surgery. In addition, there should be a clear understanding of the intracranial pathology as well as the issues associated with it during anesthesia and surgery. This understanding is essential for proper planning and management of the case. All potential problems, such as airway management, intravenous (IV) line sites, central line sites, and patency of radial artery, should be addressed.[3]

Neurosurgical patients should have 2 peripheral IV lines, one reserved for medication administration and the other for volume management. Moreover, it may be beneficial to insert a central venous catheter if the case indicates it. Cases that would indicate placement of a central line would be cases that the surgeon anticipates a large blood loss or fluid shifts. A central line would allow the anesthetist to rapidly transfuse fluids, blood products, and vasoactive medications to an unstable patient. The central line is helpful to the neuro-anesthetist for monitoring and trending central venous pressures that can be used to guide intravascular volume status and for administering potent cardiovascular medications. Mannitol, which is a commonly used osmotic diuretic, is used for acute control of increased ICP.[3] Mannitol pulls water from the brain and tissues into the intravascular space.[1] However, mannitol can cause local inflammation on injection when administered through a peripheral IV. Administering large or frequent doses of mannitol through a central line is preferable and decreases the local inflammation.[3]

The topic of premedication for a neurosurgical procedure is up for debate. Certain premedications, such as narcotics, should be avoided. Narcotics cause a decrease in respiratory drive, which leads to an increase in $Paco_2$, resulting in an increase in cerebral blood flow and cerebral blood volume.[4] Increased cerebral blood flow and cerebral blood volume may be harmful to neurosurgical patients, especially to patients with aneurysmal subarachnoid hemorrhage.[4] However, many patients may benefit from a benzodiazepine before the induction of anesthesia to decrease their anxiety level.

If the case is an emergency, an abbreviated preoperative evaluation will need to be completed, including major health problems, past surgeries, neurologic status, airway assessment, allergies, last oral intake, and adequate IV access.

INDUCTION CONSIDERATION

Induction of anesthesia is a critical period of time because of the extremely stimulating effects of direct laryngoscopy and intubation. These events can lead to hypertension, tachycardia, and increased ICP. Induction may be followed a short time later with pinning of the head for optimal positioning in certain cases. Pinning of the head can be very painful and involves the surgeon securing the head to a headrest with screws. The anesthetists must anticipate this painful stimulus to prevent any sudden increases in heart rate or blood pressure.[1] During induction, various noxious stimuli, such as laryngoscopy and intubation, suctioning, coughing, skeletal fixation of the head or pinning, may produce a sudden increase in blood pressure, which can be harmful and must be treated quickly.

There are various types of inductions of anesthesia, including IV induction, inhalational induction, and rapid sequence induction. An IV induction is the most common and preferred method of induction for neurosurgical procedures.[4] The most common induction agent of choice is propofol. If patients are hemodynamically unstable, etomidate or ketamine can be used. Etomidate and ketamine do not cause the significant hypotension that propofol does. Etomidate is an IV induction agent that has minimal cardiorespiratory depression.[3] In addition, etomidate reduces ICP and cerebral blood flow.[3] Any of these medications are acceptable as long as they are carefully titrated to prevent any acute changes in blood pressure, which can lead to increased ICP with hypertension and decreased cerebral blood flow with significant hypotension.[4] Opioids, such as fentanyl or remifentanil infusion, are also used.[4] For muscle relaxation, which is necessary for endotracheal intubation, either succinylcholine or a nondepolarizing muscle relaxant can be administered. There has been some discussions about using succinylcholine in patients with elevated ICP; however, it is noted the possible effects of increased ICP are usually quick and can be mitigated by increasing patients' anesthetic depth with some additional propofol.[1]

Neuromuscular blockade may not be necessary throughout the surgery but should be used during positioning and head stabilization.[1] Data support pretreatment with lidocaine to minimize elevation in ICP as well as the defasciculation dose of a nondepolarizing muscle relaxant if succinylcholine is to be used.[1] In addition, the increase in ICP previously observed with the administration of succinylcholine is avoided when patients are deeply anesthetized or when a defasculating dose of a nondepolarizing muscle relaxant is given. However, using a nondepolarizing muscle relaxant, such as rocuronium, may be a better choice.[4]

Preoxygenation for 3 to 5 minutes before induction is common practice.[3] Accurate airway management is vital to prevent the dual insults of hypoxia and hypercarbia. After patients are intubated, the endotracheal tube is verified by auscultation and the presence of end tidal carbon dioxide. The endotracheal tube is then secured, and the eyes are taped for protection. Patients are then positioned; pressure points are protected, and acute flexion of the neck is avoided. As previously mentioned, before skeletal traction is applied additional doses of propofol or fentanyl can be given to prevent a hypertensive crisis.

INTRAOPERATIVE CONSIDERATIONS
Positioning Concerns

Positioning a patient for a surgical procedure requires all surgical team members to work as a group to ensure patient safety. The goal of patient positioning is nerve injury prevention, while providing the surgeon with optimum operating conditions.[3] Postoperative peripheral nerve injury is frequently ascribed to incorrect surgical positioning, whereas perioperative nerve injury can be associated with positioning devices. The degree of risk when positioning surgical patients is amplified when an anesthetic is administered. Anesthetized patients are rendered incapable of making changes in their position when needed.[3]

Supine

The supine position is the most common of all surgical positions. When supine, the patients' head remains neutral or turned left or right for frontal, parietal, or temporal access. When these extreme changes in head positioning occur, jugular venous drainage is impeded. Patients undergoing bifrontal craniotomies and transsphenoidal techniques to the pituitary are usually maintained in the head neutral position.[5]

Prone

Patients undergoing procedures involving the spinal cord, posterior fossa, or occipital lobe are placed in the prone position. In the prone position, the neck is flexed, with the operating room (OR) table in reverse Trendelenburg, and legs elevated. The head is fixed within a pin holder, foam headrest, or horseshoe headrest.[5]

Additional goals with patients positioned prone include prevention of inferior vena cava compression. Impaired blood flow through the vena cava redirects blood to the epidural plexus and increases the risk for bleeding during surgery. Although reducing vena cava pressure is a goal of all spinal surgery OR tables, although infrequent, they can increase the risk of air embolism.[5]

Sitting

Surgeons use the sitting position when access to midline structures is required. Patients are positioned in a modified recumbent position as opposed to a true sitting position. The legs are elevated to promote venous return.[5] Cardiovascular changes in the sitting position include decreases in cardiac output and blood pressure when extremities are positioned below the level of the heart. Patients in the sitting position who become hypotensive may be at an increased risk for hypoperfusion and ischemia.[3] The sitting position has several benefits in comparison with the supine position. The sitting position aids in reducing both ICP and blood loss, while preserving cranial nerve function. The major risks involving the sitting position include venous air embolism, postprocedure incidence of pneumocephalus, subdural hematoma, tetraplegia, macroglossia, and peripheral nerve injury.[6]

Padding

Protective padding, although an integral component of patient positioning, when used improperly can increase a patient's risk for perioperative nerve injury. Despite documenting the use of padding at the elbow, 27% of cases by Welch and colleagues[7] developed an ulnar nerve injury. Any surgical position can compromise normal respiratory or cardiovascular physiology. The type of anesthetic administered, patient comorbidities, and body habitus can enhance these physiologic changes. When positioning any patient, attention to the disruption of normal physiologic changes should be considered during the planning, implementation, and return to his or her baseline supine position. Prevention is key to lessening the incidence of position related injuries.[3]

Neuromonitoring

Monitoring of spinal cord motor tracts is used in spinal surgery, whereby electrical activity at the surgical site can be evaluated.[5] Monitoring of motor evoked potentials is a prognosticator of a patient's postoperative motor function.[3] This method of monitoring allows the neurophysiologist to assess the integrity of the corticospinal and corticobulbar tract while patients are anesthetized.[3]

Intracranial Pressure Management

The normal ICP is usually 5 to 15 mm Hg. If an increase were to occur in one portion of intracranial volume, there must be a simultaneous decrease in another portion to avert an increase in ICP.[8] Techniques used to reduce an elevated ICP include raising the head of the bed if the surgery allows, increasing ventilation, draining cerebrospinal fluid (CSF), administering hyperosmotic medications, administering diuretics, or administering steroids. The anesthetist can also administer anesthetic medications, such as barbiturates and propofol, that can cause cerebral vasoconstriction. In addition, the surgeon can decompress the area, which would require excellent communication between the surgeon and anesthesia team.[8]

Monitoring

Standard monitoring for neurosurgical procedures includes electrocardiogram, blood pressure measurement by both cuff and arterial line, pulse oximetry, inspired oxygen concentration, end-tidal carbon dioxide, temperature, Foley catheter, precordial stethoscope, and neuromonitoring if required.[3]

Maintenance

During the maintenance phase of the anesthetic, the head of the OR table is usually elevated 15° to 30° to promote venous and CSF drainage. The head may be turned to one side or the other to optimize surgical exposure. If the neck is flexed, it will interfere with venous drainage and increase ICP.

Anesthetic techniques can vary from an oxygen-air-narcotic technique, inhalational agent, or a total IV anesthetic technique with propofol. Once intubation has occurred, end-tidal carbon dioxide levels ($ETCO_2$) should be kept between 30 and 35 mm Hg and verified through arterial blood gases. $ETCO_2$ is monitored to evaluate and ensure adequate ventilation throughout the case. Normothermia should be maintained throughout the procedure.[3]

Brain Relaxation Techniques

Patients presenting to the OR with a brain mass can exhibit symptoms of increased ICP secondary to brain tissue swelling. An enlarged brain makes tumor removal complicated. In order to reduce brain swelling and tumor removal, steps are taken to diminish brain swelling. This technique is known as brain relaxation.[9] Medication, such as mannitol or hypertonic saline solution, can be given as a medical management to provide brain relaxation for craniotomies that require opening of the dura mater. This therapy is called hyperosmolar therapy and is important to use in patients with intracranial hypertension.[9]

Fluids

Throughout the course of a neurosurgical procedure, fluid requirements are closely monitored. Preoperative fluid deficits and intraoperative blood and fluid losses must be replaced. Close monitoring of fluid administration minimizes the incidence of cerebral edema, elevated ICP, diminished cerebral perfusion pressure, and ischemia. Fluids that contain sodium are administered to maintain perfusion and prevent hypovolemia.[3]

SURGERY SPECIFIC CONSIDERATIONS
Craniotomy for Elective Aneurysm Clipping

Elective aneurysm intervention decreases patients' chances of rebleeding. Rebleeding is the primary cause of patient mortality. Postclipping vasospasm can occur and is treated with volume loading and induced hypotension. Elective clipping also decreases hospitalization and other postprocedure complications that include deep vein thrombosis, atelectasis, and pneumonia.[3] Anesthesia considerations include avoiding hypertension, brain relaxation, maintaining a normal to high mean arterial blood pressure (MAP), and the ability to accomplish specific MAP control. Monitors include an arterial line and a central venous pressure catheter if needed. An anesthetic technique that enables acceptable control of the MAP and prevents hypertension is a requirement for the care of these patients.[3]

Craniotomy for Subdural Hematoma

Subdural hematomas occur when veins tear and leak into the subdural space primarily from head trauma and are verified by computed tomography scan. Geriatric patients may have sustained head trauma and do not remember it. Presenting symptoms may include headache and drowsiness that can vary from hour to hour. Patients may also experience other neurologic findings, such as hemiparesis and language difficulties. Geriatric patients may also experience symptoms of dementia.[8]

Individuals whose condition has stabilized may benefit from conservative medical treatment; however, surgical clot evacuation is preferable for most patients. Surgical evacuation of a subdural hematoma can be performed through burr holes under general, local, or sedation as methods of anesthesia. If the subdural is chronic or contains clotted blood, a craniotomy would be required.[8]

Spines

Spine surgery can involve patients undergoing a microdiscectomy to multilevel fusions that are increasingly complex and lengthy. The anesthesia plan of care for these patients is complicated by the patients' age, comorbidities, and monitoring techniques.[10] Spinal cord injuries typically involve surgical intervention for decompression of the spinal cord for patients with neurologic impairment in hopes of restoring the spinal column alignment as well as spinal stability.[10] Anesthesia providers are responsible for multiple aspects of care, which include managing the airway, intraoperative care, and resuscitation.[10]

Many spine cases involve patients positioned prone on the OR table. Complicated procedures involve multiple levels, instrumentation, and large fluid losses. Hardware placed by surgeons can also injure the spinal cord. Spine procedures are also performed for tumor resection, hematomas, or abscess drainage.[11]

EMERGENCE FROM ANESTHESIA
Considerations

If the plan is to extubate patients at the conclusion of the procedure, the anesthetic drugs should be appropriately tapered as the scalp is sutured. If fentanyl or sufentanil have been used as an infusion agent, they can be discontinued at dural closure. Remifentanil should be continued until scalp closure, and a longer-acting analgesic can be given, such as fentanyl.[1]

The ideal outcome at the conclusion of the case would be patients responding to verbal commands in order to perform a neurologic assessment.[4] Some possible guidelines for emergence include not reversing the muscle relaxant until the head dressing is applied and there is total control of the airway. All suctioning must be completed before patients receive a reversal dosage. Esmolol or labetalol can be used to treat large increases in blood pressure.[4] It is important to prevent and manage hypertension during emergence, as this has been linked to postoperative hematoma formation.[12] Once patients are hemodynamically stable and have a stable airway, they can be transferred to the intensive care unit (ICU) or postanesthesia care unit with supplemental oxygen.

Complications

A potentially devastating complication after neurosurgery is postoperative nausea and vomiting. Postoperative nausea and vomiting is an upsetting, unwanted, complex, and potentially dangerous complication because of the chance of increased ICP and cerebral intravascular pressure, which could lead to brain swelling and bleeding.[2] Postoperative nausea is especially a problem in posterior fossa forgery. Postoperative nausea and vomiting can be best treated with a multimodal approach often including ondansetron, droperidol, dexamethasone, metoclopramide, and scopolamine as well as adequate hydration.[12] Administering dexamethasone has been shown to decrease postoperative nausea and vomiting by 25%.[12]

Postoperative vision loss is another distressing complication of neurosurgery, more specifically, spine surgery. Postoperative vision loss after spinal surgery is estimated to be between 0.028% and 0.2%.[13] Postoperative vision loss is rather uncommon, but it can be a life-changing complication for patients. In addition, it has an unknown origin and pathogenesis.[13] Besides spinal surgery, postoperative vision loss has also been known to occur after coronary artery bypass surgery, craniotomy, laparotomy, radical neck dissection, hip arthroplasty, and lumber surgery.[13] Some variables thought to contribute to the development of postoperative vision loss include intraoperative hypotension, length of surgery, amount of blood loss, use of crystalloid and colloids for fluid replacement, and anemia. The most significant variable in developing postoperative vision loss is long length of surgery, large volume of blood loss, and large amounts of replacement fluids administered.[13]

Postoperative Management

Some important postoperative factors to keep in mind are fluid and electrolyte balance and fluid management. Diuretics are frequently used intraoperatively to decrease ICP and to facilitate intracranial dissection. Mannitol is associated with significant potassium urinary excretion as well as volume and electrolyte shifts that have to be managed in the postoperative period. This complication results in a higher risk of cardiac arrhythmias that need to be monitored in the ICU.[2]

Postoperative analgesia is a very important topic in neuro-anesthesia. It has been shown that inadequate pain control can cause discomfort and may lead to increased postoperative complications and prolonged hospital stay. The current practice for postoperative management in craniotomies is a multimodal approach that includes scalp blocks with local anesthetics, nonsteroidal antiinflammatories, and opioids.[2] Patient-controlled analgesia can be used; however, sedative opioids would be used cautiously in these patients. Opioids can have effects on neurologic function and cognitive abilities; this can impair the clinical evaluation in order to detect acute changes in neurologic status.[2]

CONSIDERATIONS FOR THE INTENSIVE CARE UNIT NURSE

When moving patients directly from the OR to the ICU, one of the most important aspects is the transfer of care. The transfer of care and report handoff is very important to maintain excellent patient care and safety. If something critical is not mentioned in the report, it can lead to improper care of patients.[14]

Another consideration for the intensive care nurse is the importance of frequent neurologic examinations to quickly detect any changes in patients' status. The nurse needs to monitor patients' neurologic status, hemodynamic status, fluid and electrolytes status, as well as manage postoperative pain. Patients will require frequent vital signs and neurologic monitoring immediately postoperatively. Urine output, electrolytes, and fluid balance need to be assessed. Dressings and surgical incisions require periodic assessment to detect any increased bleeding at the incision site or hematomas. A challenging consideration for the ICU nurse is to keep patients comfortable and calm in the immediate postoperative period. If there is concern for increased ICP in a particular patient, the nurse may have to stager his or her interventions to allow the patient to rest and the ICP to return to baseline. For example, patients may have to tolerate being turned and suctioned in a short period of time. Taking care of neurosurgical patients requires attentiveness and focus to allow the nurse to pick up subtle changes in the patients' status.[14]

REFERENCES

1. Chander D, Gelb AW. Anaesthesia for neurosurgery. In: Evidence-based anaesthesia and intensive care. 2006. p. 282.
2. Bilotta F, Guerra C, Rosa G. Update on anesthesia for craniotomy. Curr Opin Anaesthesiol 2013;26:517–22.
3. Nagelhout JJ, Plaus KL. Nurse anesthesia. 5th edition. St Louis (MI): Elsevier Saunders; 2014.
4. Kundra S, Mahendru V, Choudhary AK. Principles of neuroanesthesia in aneurysmal subarachnoid hemorrhage. J Anaesthesiol Clin Pharmacol 2014;30: 328–37.
5. Miller RD, Eriksson LI, Fleisher LA, et al. Miller's anesthesia, 2 volume set. 8th edition. 2015. Available at: www.elsevier.com.
6. Gracia I, Fabregas N. Craniotomy in sitting position: anesthesiology management. Curr Opin Anaesthesiol 2014;27(5):474–83.
7. Welch MB, Walsh CM, Tremper TD, et al. Perioperative peripheral nerve injuries. Anesthesiology 2009;111:490–7.
8. Hines RL, Marschall KE. Stoelting's anesthesia and co-existing disease. 6th edition. Philadelphia: Elsevier Saunders; 2012.
9. Prabhakar H, Singh GP, Anand V, et al. Mannitol versus hypertonic saline for brain relaxation in patients undergoing craniotomy. Sao Paulo Med J 2015;133:166–7.
10. Barash PG, Cullen BF, Stoelting RK, et al. Clinical anesthesia. 7th edition. Philadelphia: Wolters Kluwer; 2013.
11. Butterworth JF, Mackey DC, Wasnick JD. Morgan & Mikhail's clinical anesthesiology. 5th edition. New York: McGraw Hill; 2013.
12. Dinsmore J. Anaesthesia for elective neurosurgery. Br J Anaesth 2007;99:68–74.
13. Baig MN, Lubow M, Immesocte P, et al. Vision loss after spine surgery: review of the literature and recommendations. Neurosurg Focus 2007;23(5):1–9.
14. Ong M, Coiera E. Handoff and care transitions. In: Agrawal A, editor. Patient safety a care based comprehensive guide. 2014. p. 35–51. http://dx.doi.org/10.1007/978-14614-7419-7_3.

Optic Nerve Sheath Diameter Ultrasound and the Diagnosis of Increased Intracranial Pressure

Christopher Hylkema, MSN, RN, CEN, CFRN*

KEYWORDS

- Ultrasound • ICP • Optic nerve sheath diameter

KEY POINTS

- Optic nerve sheath diameter ultrasound is a safe, valid, and noninvasive method of measuring intracranial pressure (ICP) with high sensitivity and specificity.
- The procedure is simple and easily learned by experienced and nonexperienced clinicians.
- Implications for providers include rapid diagnosis of elevated ICP and early medical and surgical intervention.
- Optic nerve sheath diameter ultrasound has a possible role as a screening tool for increased ICP in the patient with neurologic compromise.

Increased intracranial pressure (ICP) is a common phenomenon in the neurocritically ill patient with traumatic brain injury. The sequelae of increased ICP can cause severe disability or death if not recognized and managed immediately.[1–4] In the United States alone, more than 53,000 individuals succumb to traumatic brain injury–related deaths.[5] This amount accounts for 30.5% of all injury-related deaths and is estimated to cost the health care system approximately 76.5 billion dollars a year.[5] After an initial insult, such as blunt or penetrating trauma to the head, an increase in blood volume or edema may cause a rising pressure in the rigid inflexible vault that is the skull. These patients and their presentations are noted to be highly time-sensitive and present to emergency rooms with poor examination, limited history, or other clinical information.[5] Earlier diagnosis of elevated ICP after a traumatic event can allow for faster temporizing measures and definitive treatment in the neurologically compromised patient and improved outcomes.[5]

Although direct ventriculostomy is considered to be the gold standard of measuring ICP, the procedure is invasive, poses risks to the patient, and often is traditionally only

The author has no conflicts of interest to disclose.
Thomas Jefferson University Hospital, Thomas Jefferson University, Philadelphia, PA, USA
* 111 South 11th Street, Philadelphia, PA 19107.
E-mail address: christopher.hylkema@jefferson.edu

performed by trained neurosurgeons. Lumbar punctures can also be used to diagnose elevated ICP. However, lumbar punctures carry risks as well, such as infection or bleeding, and can be time and resource intensive if performed on a critically ill patient. Their success can be hindered by many factors, such as body habitus, spinal hardware, or user skill. In addition, if there is obstructive hydrocephalus or concern for a compressing intracranial lesion, the lumbar puncture may not be the procedure of choice.

Other modalities such as computed tomography (CT) imaging can be done rapidly and relatively inexpensively. However, repeated CT scans expose patients to large doses of radiation and frequently require the nurse to travel with the patient, even with the increasing prevalence of portable CT scanners. In addition, traditional markers of increased ICP on CT scan, such as midline shift, basal cistern, and sulcal effacement, may not reliably confirm increased ICP.[6] MRI provides high-quality images, but is labor intensive, time intensive on the part of the nursing staff, or is not appropriate for routine assessment of increased ICPs, and many patients cannot be put in the MRI machine or are too hemodynamically unstable for MRI.

An ideal neuromonitoring tool in the neurocritically ill would be readily available, easily performed by nonradiologists, is rapid, and is noninvasive. Such technology exists today and is available in almost every intensive care unit (ICU) and emergency department in the United States—the portable ultrasound. Ultrasound can be used to measure ICP through a transorbital evaluation.

Ultrasound has been used since the early 1980s to assist clinicians in the diagnosis and clinical decision-making of critically ill patients.[7] Although ultrasound is now considered to be a standard of care in emergency and critical care medicine, machine cost and size and training have historically limited their utility. The advent of smaller, lighter, and more durable ultrasound machines has heralded the use of sonography in many emergency departments, ICUs, and even the prehospital environment with great success.[7]

This article discusses the optic nerve sheath diameter (ONSD) ultrasound procedure and highlights current literature that supports its validity and its implications to advanced practice providers.

SUMMARY OF PROCEDURE

In patients with increased ICP, physical examination findings can often be limited due to decreased responsiveness, being intubated, or being paralyzed. It is well documented that examination findings in the eye can reflect conditions elsewhere in the body. In the setting of increased ICP, papilledema, or swelling of the optic nerve disc, can take hours before it is clinically appreciated.[8] ONSD ultrasound, however, can be performed and can detect these changes in ICP before they are appreciated on physical examination. The optic nerve sheath attaches to the globe on the posterior aspect. The optic nerve sheath is contiguous with the dura mater and has an arachnoid space in which cerebrospinal fluid percolates.[8] As ICP increases, this optic nerve sheath space swells and can be appreciated on ultrasound. A typical optic nerve sheath is less than 5 mm. A finding greater than this may correlate with an ICP greater than 20 mm Hg.[8]

To perform the study, one needs an ultrasound machine with a high-frequency linear probe. The probe is placed on the patient's closed eye. Many clinicians may use a tegaderm to prevent ultrasound gel from getting in the eye. A view of the globe can be obtained. The optic nerve sheath appears as a darkened, vertical, linear pattern approximately 3 mm posterior to the globe. The clinician can then measure the diameter of this line. If it is greater than 5 mm, it is 100% correlated with an ICP greater than 20 mm Hg. The literature also suggests that as ICP increases, ONSD increases in a linear fashion.[9] Because of the simple nature of the examination and the limited time needed to perform it, it is an ideal test for emergency clinicians to evaluate patients with change in mental status of unknown cause and to initiate time-sensitive, often life-saving interventions directed at reducing ICP.[9]

Review of the Literature

Amini and colleagues[10,11] used a descriptive prospective study to compare 50 nontrauma patients, who, for various different diagnoses, were candidates for lumbar puncture. Sonography was performed; immediately after, the lumbar puncture was initiated. Correlation tests were used, and using an optimum characteristic curve, the value of 20 cmH$_2$O was set to define elevated ICP. In patients with ICP less than 20 cmH$_2$O, the mean ONSD was 4.60 mm. Those with elevated ICPs had a mean ONSD of 6.6 mm. The study concluded that ONSD greater than 5.5 predicted ICP greater than 20 cmH$_2$O with 100% sensitivity and specificity. The researchers found that ONSD is a strong predictor of increased ICP, and ultrasound may be considered highly useful as a screening tool so that prompt therapeutic interventions can be instituted due to its availability, fast application, and high sensitivity. Although the population size was somewhat limited, the study shows a strong diagnostic comparison of ultrasound of the ONSD and the lumbar puncture procedure in diagnosing elevated ICP.

Dubourg and colleagues[6] sought to perform a comprehensive analysis of the diagnostic accuracy of ultrasound of the ONSD. They performed a review, without language restriction, that included electronic databases as well as a manual review of literature and conference proceedings. Data were extracted independently by 3 investigators, and they performed random effects meta-analysis and metaregression. After reviewing 699 articles, 675 articles were excluded after reviewing their abstracts. From there, 24 were selected for full review, and subsequently, 6 articles were chosen for the meta-analysis. The investigators included 6 cross-sectional studies involving a total of 231 patients. In each study, sensitivity and specificity (comparing ICP via ventriculostomy and ultrasound of ONSD) were compared. The pooled sensitivity in this study was determined to be 90%. That would suggest that up to 10% of patients with increased ICP may go undetected. The investigators assert that due to the severe nature of neurocritical illness, a missed diagnosis of increased ICP can be catastrophic. ONSD ultrasound, therefore, should be used in conjunction with other methods such as imaging to confirm diagnosis. Because of these limitations, the investigators assert that ONSD ultrasound should not be used alone for diagnosis if other means are available. It may be of utility when direct ICP monitoring is contraindicated or unavailable. The investigators self-identify the study's limitations in including only 6 studies. These investigators also identify ultrasound of the ONSD as a valuable screening tool and assert that it may be useful in the ICU for intermittent monitoring and diagnosis. Furthermore, they speculate that in the emergency setting it may be helpful for determining whether physicians at small or community hospitals should maintain the patient at their facility or transfer them to higher-level tertiary care centers for the placement of an invasive device.

Frumin and colleagues[12–15] performed a blinded observational study involving 27 patients admitted to a level 1 trauma center. The patients all required ventriculostomy placement and ICP monitoring. The study used one trained sonographer to perform ONSD ultrasounds on each of the patients within 24 hours of external ventricular drain (EVD) placement. This study also used the cutoff of 20 cmH$_2$O and ONSD of greater than or equal to 5.2 mm to define elevated ICP. The sonographic measurements yielded 83.3% sensitivity and 100% specificity for diagnosing intracranial hypertension when compared with invasive ICP monitoring. The study further asserted that the expansion of the ONSD is predictable; however, it may not follow a linear pattern. The investigators do not think that ONSD will replace EVDs and ICP monitoring; however, they assert that ultrasound has the potential to diagnose increased ICP when other means are unavailable, incurs no harm to the patient, and provides a simple, noninvasive method of measuring ICP.

Implications for Clinicians

As clinicians tasked with performing diagnosis and initiation of treatment, it is important to recognize the potential as well as the limitations of this procedure. It is suggested that clinicians who have used ultrasound before may be able to learn how to accurately perform the study after performing it on only 10 patients with 3 abnormal ICP scan results.[6] Users who are unfamiliar with ultrasound may need to perform closer to 25 scans to accurately assess ONSD.[6]

Despite the potential of this procedure (international guidelines still suggest that patients with traumatic brain injury and a Glasgow coma scale less than 8 should receive invasive ICP monitoring), ultrasound is not a panacea. Clinicians should also be aware that time from admission to hospital to ventriculostomy placement is often greater than 1 hour.[6] ONSD ultrasound may fill this gap because it can be performed in the interim and allow for earlier management.

With findings of increased ICP, clinicians direct their therapy at reducing ICP, controlling cerebral perfusion pressure, and reducing the cerebral metabolism of the brain. These measures, however, are usually temporizing in conjunction with, or until, definitive surgical management such as hemicraniotomy can be performed. Although an in-depth discussion of the merits of 3% sodium chloride versus mannitol exceeds the scope of this article, osmotic diuretics and loop diuretic agents such as lasix, ethracrynic acid, create an osmotic gradient and shift fluid away from the brain.[16,17] Propofol, phenobarbital, and sodium thiopental are hypnotic and barbiturate agents that are used to reduce cerebral metabolism and oxygen consumption,[16] reduce cerebral blood flow, and subsequently ICP, and may be neuroprotective in allowing neural cells to withstand decreased cerebral perfusion pressure.[16]

SUMMARY

The expanding role of clinicians such as advanced practice nurses offers increased opportunities for research to demonstrate their ability to learn and perform these procedures with diagnostic accuracy. The investigators above discuss the importance of further research involving performance comparison studies involving clinical imaging modalities. Many of the articles reviewed also identify the need for larger studies with increased scientific rigor. Furthermore, patients with ocular trauma or abnormality are excluded from studies including the meta-analysis, and these populations may be considered in future work.

In summary, ultrasound of the ONSD is a safe, noninvasive, and accurate predictor of increased ICP. Although not a new procedure, it appears to have an underutilized application in the neurocritical care population. There is a robust body of literature to suggest its utility in patients with traumatic brain injury and patients with nontraumatic abnormality. Clinicians may be able to use this as a screening tool for increased ICP, to initiate early treatment, and to monitor the effectiveness of treatment in conjunction with other imaging modalities and invasive monitoring when available and appropriate. Treatment should be directed at temporizing measures such as pharmacologic and ventilator and surgical strategies to reduce ICP to promote better outcomes.

REFERENCES

1. Pickard J, Czosnyka M. Management of raised intracranial pressure. J Neurol Neurosurg Psychiatr 1993;56:845–58.
2. Price DD, Wilson SR, Murphy TG. Trauma ultrasound feasibility during helicopter transport. Air Med J 2000;19(4):144–6.
3. Sayed M, Zagharani E. Prehospital emergency ultrasound: a review of current clinical applications, challenges, and future implications. Emerg Med Int 2013; 2013:531674.
4. Sippel S, Muruganandan K, Levine A, et al. Review article: use of ultrasound in the developing world. Int J Emerg Med 2011;4:72.
5. Alali AS, Fowler RA, Mainprize TG, et al. Intracranial pressure monitoring in severe traumatic brain injury: results from the American College of Surgeons trauma quality improvement program. J Neurotrauma 2013;30:1–10.
6. Dubourg J, Javouhey E, Geeraerts T, et al. Ultrasonography of optic nerve sheath diameter for detection of raised intracranial pressure: a systematic review and meta-analysis. Intensive Care Med 2011;37:1059.
7. Nelson BP, Chason K. Use of ultrasound by emergency medical services: a review. Int J Emerg Med 2008;1(4):253–9.
8. Adhikari S. Ocular ultrasound. 2008. Available at: http://www.sonoguide.com/smparts_ocular.html. Accessed November 2, 2015.
9. Cotton J. Keeping an eye on increased intracranial pressure: measuring ICP using ultrasound. 2012. Available at: http://ukemig-quickhit.com/2012/10/15/keeping-an-eye-on-intracranial-pressure-measuring-icp-using-ocular-ultrasound/. Accessed November 2, 2015.
10. Amini A, Kariman H, Dolatabadi AA, et al. Use of the sonographic diameter of optic nerve sheath to estimate intracranial pressure. Am J Emerg Med 2013;31: 236–9.
11. Calvert N, Hind D, McWilliams R, et al. Ultrasound for central venous cannulation: economic evaluation of cost-effectiveness. Anaesthesia 2004;59(11):1116–20.
12. Frumin E, Schlang J, Wiechmann W, et al. Prospective analysis of single operator sonographic optic nerve sheath diameter measurement for diagnosis of elevated intracranial pressure. West J Emerg Med 2014;15(2):217–20.
13. Hansen H-C, Lagereze W, Krueger O, et al. Dependence of the optic nerve sheath diameter on acutely applied subarachnoidal pressure—an experimental ultrasound study. Acta Opthalmol 2011;89(6):e528–32.
14. Kalantari H, Jaiswal R, Bruck I, et al. Correlation of optic nerve sheath diameter measurements by computed tomography and magnetic resonance imaging. Am J Emerg Med 2013;31(11):1595–7.
15. Melanson S, Mccarthy J, Stromski CJ, et al. Aeromedical trauma sonography by flight crews with a miniature ultrasound unit. Prehosp Emerg Care 2001;5(4): 399–402.
16. Winkler S. Pharmacotherapy of increased ICP. 1998. Available at: http://www.uic.edu/classes/pmpr/pmpr652/Final/Winkler/ICP.html. Accessed November 2, 2015.
17. Yeager S, Doust C, Epting S, et al. Embrace Hope: an end-of-life intervention to support neurological critical care patients and their families. Crit Care Nurse 2010;30(1):47–58.

The Use of Automated Pupillometry in Critical Care

DaiWai M. Olson, RN, PhD, CCRN*, Megan Fishel, RN, BSN, CCRN

KEYWORDS

- Multimodal monitoring • Neurologic assessment • Pupillometer
- Cranial nerve assessment

KEY POINTS

- The pupillary light reflex assessment evaluates the functional ability of the optic and oculomotor cranial nerves.
- Subjective (observational) scoring of the size, shape, and reactivity of the pupil in response to light is associated with limited interrater reliability.
- Thermometer technology replaced hand-to-skin temperature assessment. Objective scoring with automated pupillometry is a natural progression in technology.
- Although there is no consensus for which parameters are of most importance, the maximum size and neuropupillary index (NPi) are most frequently documented.
- The ability to evaluate the pupillary reflex from only 1 eye at a time is a recognized limitation.

 Video content accompanies this article at http://www.ccnursing.theclinics.com/

INTRODUCTION

In romance literature, the eyes are said to be the windows to the soul. However, in the critical care setting, romance is not the issue. When performing a neurologic examination (neuroexamination) the eyes (more specifically the pupils) are closely examined, and the pupillary assessment becomes a window through which staff evaluate neurologic status. To be more specific, staff evaluate the functional status of the second cranial nerve (CN II) and third cranial nerve (CN III). This evaluation is important because

---

Disclosures: None.
The University of Texas Southwestern, Dallas, TX, USA
* Corresponding author. The University of Texas Southwestern, 5323 Harry Hines Boulevard, Dallas, TX 75390-8897.
E-mail address: DaiWai.Olson@UTSouthwestern.edu

loss of CN reflexes may signal increased intracranial pressure (ICP) and an increased risk of central brain herniation.

NEUROLOGIC EXAMINATION

Assessment is at the core of the nursing process. Performing a comprehensive neurologic examination (neuroexamination) is a cornerstone of high-quality nursing care for patients with a wide variety of neurologic and neurosurgical injuries.[1,2] The essential elements of the neuroexamination include an evaluation of level of consciousness (LOC), cognitive ability, CN function, motor function, and sensory function. By tradition, the neuroexamination is performed serially depending on the condition of the patient (eg, hourly following acute stroke). Results from each examination are compared with previous examination findings.[1,3] The results of the neuroexamination provide data that practitioners can use to formulate new treatment plans and to evaluate the impact of prior treatments.[3]

The ability of a practitioner to link the results from one element of the neuroexamination with the functional ability of a corresponding region in the central nervous system (CNS) gives rise to the concept of functional neuroanatomy. Different elements of the neuroexamination provide insight into how well specific anatomic regions of the CNS are performing. For example, changes in the LOC may provide the examiner with clues about the general function of the reticular activating system and cerebral cortex, or paresthesia of the right arm may provide clues to a left middle cerebral artery stroke.[4,5]

Nursing theory helps to define the importance of the neuroexamination to provide cues. The Coma-Cue Framework describes a paradigm whereby nurses are able to obtain cues from numerous sources of assessment and observation of patients with brain injury.[6] These cues are vital for directing nurses, and ultimately the entire health care team, toward optimally timing care interventions. The cues from a neuroexamination help guide practitioners to decide when to intervene, or allow rest, or alter a course of therapy.

During the past 50 years, a variety of assessment tools have been developed to improve the consistency with which the neuroexamination is performed, documented, and discussed. During the same half-century, numerous practice patterns have become engrained. Consciousness is most often evaluated as the patient's level of wakefulness or responsiveness to stimuli. Tools such as the Glasgow Coma Scale (GCS) and the Full Outline of Unresponsiveness (FOUR) score have been developed and refined to help guide examiners.[7-9] Portions of the GCS and FOUR score evaluate the LOC, portions evaluate the motor and sensory functions (frontal lobe, parietal lobe, thalamus), and portions evaluate some aspect of the brainstem (primarily FOUR score). A primary difference between the GCS and FOUR score is the inclusion of corneal reflexes as well as breathing pattern. Pupillary and corneal reflexes are assessed routinely as part of the CN examination. Elements of the motor and sensory examination are performed sequentially with a reflex hammer. The use of a penlight or flashlight has particularly aided CN assessment.

CRANIAL NERVES

The full assessment of CN function is an established norm that is well within the practice domain of both nurses and physicians.[1,10] The concept of functional neuroanatomy introduced earlier helps to establish the importance of linking the results of the CN examination with a specific anatomic location within the brainstem. In brief, the 12 pairs of CN roots are located throughout the brainstem. Note that although

CN I and CN II emerge from the forebrain, whereas CN III and CN IV emerge from the midbrain, CN function and anatomy are generally discussed as brainstem function.[1,11] Hence, it is convenient to discuss CN anatomy as 3 sets of 4 CNs. The first set, CN I to CN IV, emerge from the midbrain. The second set of 4, CN V to CN VII, emerges from the pons. The third set of 4, CN IX to CN XII, emerges from the medulla.[11]

Examining the pupil (pupillary light reflex) provides nurses and physicians with information about the functional status of the optic (CN II) and the oculomotor (CN III) CNs. CN II is a tract of secondary sensory pathways. The CN II pathway begins when light enters the pupil and is converted into an electrical signal by rods and cones in the retina. This signal is passed to the primary neuron (bipolar cells). The signal is then passed to ganglion cells (the secondary neurons), which converge near the optic disc. The ganglion cell axons then exit the eyeball and become what is traditionally known as the optic nerve. Most of the tracts that make up the optic nerve then run through the optic chiasm and terminate in the lateral geniculate nucleus. Visual signals are then sent along the tertiary neuron to the visual cortex in the occipital lobe. However, a portion of the tracts separate before the lateral geniculate nucleus and terminate in the pretectal area of the midbrain.[12] These tracts are vital for the pupillary light reflex.

The oculomotor CN (CN III), as implied by the name, is crucial for the motor function of the eye. The somatic nucleus of CN III is in the midbrain and gives rise to somatic motor fibers. The parasympathetic fibers of CN III originate in the Edinger-Westphal nucleus. The somatic and parasympathetic fibers combine to form the CN III. Electrical signals carried along CN III cause the muscles of the eye to contract. These contractions result in movement of the eyeball and eyelid, and also are responsible for constriction of the pupil.[12]

A brief review of the pupillary light reflex helps to highlight the importance of these complex pathways. In short, bright light stimulates a signal that is carried along the afferent pathway of CN II to the tectal plate in the midbrain and then to the Edinger-Westphal nucleus (EWN). Then, efferent pathways of CN III carry the signal from the EWN to the eye; this causes the motor fibers of the eye to contract. This contraction is seen clinically as a constriction of the pupil. Because fibers from the EWN project to both eyes, light stimulus of either eye should result in constriction of both pupils.

By tradition, pupillary examinations were performed and evaluated subjectively using either a flashlight or penlight. The examiner was asked to first score the initial size (diameter) and shape (round or irregular) of the pupil. Then, after stimulating the pupil with light, the examiner was asked to score the reactivity of the pupil. Reactivity was scored either as present versus absent, or as briskly reactive versus sluggishly reactive versus nonreactive (fixed). Despite being an ingrained element of practice, the traditional method of subjective pupillary assessment has only fair to moderate interrater reliability.[13] The interrater reliability is further decreased when skill mix, training, and a large variation in light source and examination conditions are factored into the equation.[14–17] Automated pupillometry was introduced to the intensive care unit (ICU) as an alternative to the subjectivity required by human assessors.

PUPILLOMETER

The act of measuring the pupil and evaluating the pupillary light reflex has been a standard of practice for hundreds of years.[18] Before electricity the pupil was examined by candlelight. Electric light technology allowed this practice to evolve. The hand-held flashlight and pupil gauge soon found acceptance in health care. During this evolution, evaluating the size, shape, and reactivity of the pupil was a subjective task that was part of the art of medicine and nursing care. In recent decades, objective measures of pupil size and reactivity have also evolved. In 1960, the first automated pupillometry (measuring the pupil) was first described by using 16-mm film to examine pupil dilatation in response to emotional stimuli.[19] The invention of high-speed miniaturized computer processors enabled the most recent technological evolution in pupil assessment.

At its core, automated pupillometry is a series of photographic images of the pupil digitally captured and scored for change in size over time. Hand-held portable pupillometers are now widely available and represent a logical step in nursing assessment. Historically, nurses subjectively evaluated temperature by touching the forehead, blood pressure by feeling the threadiness of the pulse, and oxygenation by observing for a bluish tinge in the lips or skin. Modern technology and human ingenuity gave rise to thermometers, manometers, and oximeters. Historically, nurses subjectively evaluated pupillary response using a variety of light sources manipulated in a variety of conditions. Modern technology and human ingenuity have again provided a technological advance to objectively measure (meter) another element of the physical examination.

The use of an automated pupillary assessment device, or pupillometer, has become increasingly common for patients with neurologic injuries.[20] The NeurOptics NPi-100 and NPi-200 are perhaps the most common commercial pupillometer devices used in critical care. These are hand-held portable devices that can be used with a disposable patient shield. This device provides a variety of measures of pupil size and reactivity, including maximum size, minimum size, constriction velocity (CV), latency, and the neuropupillary index (NPi). To obtain a reading, the practitioner (registered nurse [RN] or doctor of medicine [MD]) targets the pupil by pressing a button corresponding with either the left or right eye (Video 1). When the pupil is clearly seen on the pupillometer display screen, the practitioner releases the button; this activates the device to emit a short (0.8 second) burst of light (1000 lux). The device then stores repeated images taken at more than 30 frames per second for 3.2 seconds. From these images, the pupil is digitally scored and tracked. Results from each examination are provided on an LCD (liquid crystal display) screen within a few seconds of the examination.

The maximum pupil size and minimum pupil size are measured in millimeters to the nearest 100th (eg, 3.45 mm) decimal. The CV is measured in millimeters per second and calculated as the amount of constriction (size change) divided by the duration (time in seconds) during which the pupil remains constricted. Latency is defined as the time from light stimulus until the start of constriction. The NPi is a unique new variable, derived from a set of measurements obtained in healthy volunteers.[21] The NPi ranges from 0 to 5 and is a comparison of the response of the patient to normal responses. The NPi is therefore derived by comparing output from a mathematical algorithm obtained from normal healthy volunteers. An NPi value greater than 3.0 is considered normal, whereas NPi values less than 3 are considered abnormal and associated with intracranial hypertension.[22] An NPi of zero (no pupil constriction) equates with a fixed pupil (absent pupillary reflex).

DISCUSSION

The underlying concept of the pupillometer is simply an automation of the traditional pupillary assessment. Moreover, automating measurements is not new. Pulse oximetry automates the assessment of nail bed color and is a natural extension to measure tissue perfusion. Thermometers automate the assessment of how hot or cold the forehead feels, and are the natural extension to measure temperature. Blood pressure measurement, whether invasive or noninvasive, is a natural replacement for the evaluation of how thready or robust a pulse feels to the assessor. Automating pupil assessment is therefore simply the next step in providing more consistent and reliable data from which to evaluate the patients' status.

Although it seems clear that pupillometry is an emerging technology that will become a mainstay in critical care, there are a variety of unanswered questions that require study. Can the device be used to compare the size of the left pupil with that of the right pupil (anisocoria), or is the device only useful to compare pupil reactivity? What are the normal ranges for pupillometry output data (NPi, CV, latency, pupil size), and which of these data should be documented? What are the assessment parameters that should prompt nursing action? Should readings be interpreted as absolutes, or are serial readings required? Is there a continued role for performance of the subjective examination (penlight)? The answers to these questions are likely to help to standardize practice, but will also generate new questions.

A recognized limitation of hand-held pupillometry is that the current version of the device is used to examine only 1 eye (pupil) at a time, and therefore may not provide adequate information to rule out the presence or absence of anisocoria (unequal sized pupils). Although there is no agreed-on cut point at which the pupils are deemed to be unequal in size, it is generally accepted that greater than 1.0-mm difference in pupil diameter (left eye vs right eye) is considered anisocoria.[2,23,24] Although anisocoria can be a normal finding in approximately 20% of the population, there is some evidence that the presence of anisocoria is associated with worse clinical outcomes. To be specific, the presence of anisocoria in the setting of traumatic brain injury is a sign of secondary brain injury and may herald neurologic deterioration.[25,26]

Although objective assessments provide more precise and reliable data, there is only an assumption that better data will result in better outcomes. Recent literature has examined automated pupillometry compared with subjective examination. There is inadequate interrater reliability between humans in evaluating pupil size, shape, and reactivity. In a recent study of more than 2300 paired assessments, the interrater reliability between 2 RNs, 2 MDs, or an RN and an MD was inadequate to support the assumption that any one practitioner would score pupil function the same as any other practitioner. This finding was especially noted for fixed pupils (<50% agreement that a pupil was not reactive).[13] Meeker and colleagues[27] found only limited interrater reliability for subjective scoring of size, shape, and reactivity between practitioners.

Pupillometers provide several new values that are not available with subjective assessment. Of these, NPi is the most widely reported. Several studies suggest that NPi, as a measure of pupil function, is associated with early detection of intracranial disorder.[28,29] However, there are no studies that have been designed to prospectively evaluate outcomes linked specifically to treatments that are determined by NPi data. Moreover, although an NPi of less than 3.0 is established as a general criterion for abnormal pupillary reaction, there are inadequate normative data to determine whether this relationship is linear (ie, whether an NPi of 1.0 is half as good as an NPi of 2.0). Variables such as CV, minimum size, and maximum size are intuitive to most practitioners. However, because these variables are only recently available, intuition mandates testing.

Nursing assessment is steeped in practical pearls. New ICU nurses are quickly educated that teeth brushing can mimic tachycardia, or that pulse oximetry is unreliable in the setting of carbon monoxide toxicity. Likely, there are medical and pharmaceutical conditions that will be revealed as conditions in which pupillometry should be interpreted cautiously.

SUMMARY

Hospitals across the globe are quickly adopting a practice that includes automated pupillometer assessment.[30,31] Assessment of pupillary function is a noninvasive method of providing vital information about patients' current neurologic function.[2,32] Pupil size, shape, and reactivity provides an indication of CN function for CN II and CN III, as well as providing insight into the sympathetic nervous system functional status. When optimally functional, light stimulus to 1 or both pupils causes constriction of both pupils. Given that the bilateral pathways (afferent and efferent) are intact, the normal finding is that the pupils are equal in size, round, and reactive to light. Abnormal findings are associated with specific injury such as CN III damage, and brainstem or transtentorial herniation.[33–35]

SUPPLEMENTARY DATA

Supplementary data related to this article can be found online at http://dx.doi.org/10.1016/j.cnc.2015.09.003.

REFERENCES

1. Bader MK, Littlejohns LR. AANN Core curriculum for neuroscience nursing. 5th edition. Glenview (IL): American Association of Neuroscience Nurses; 2010.
2. Campbell WW. DeJong's the neurologic examination. 7th edition. Philadelphia: Lippincott Williams & Wilkins; 2005.
3. Singhal NS, Josephson SA. A practical approach to neurologic evaluation in the intensive care unit. J Crit Care 2014;29(4):627–33.
4. Plum F, Posner JB. The diagnosis of stupor and coma. 3rd edition. Philadelphia: Davis; 1980.
5. Mazzoni P, Pearson TS, Rowland LP, et al. Merritt's neurology handbook. Philadelphia: Lippincott Williams & Wilkins; 2006.
6. Olson DM, Graffagnino C. Consciousness, coma, and caring for the brain-injured patient. AACN Clin Issues 2005;16(4):441–55.
7. Teasdale G, Jennett B. Assessment of coma and impaired consciousness. A practical scale. Lancet 1974;2(7872):81–4.
8. Wijdicks EF, Bamlet WR, Maramattom BV, et al. Validation of a new coma scale: the FOUR score. Ann Neurol 2005;58(4):585–93.
9. Iyer VN, Mandrekar JN, Danielson RD, et al. Validity of the FOUR score coma scale in the medical intensive care unit. Mayo Clin Proc 2009;84(8):694–701.
10. Greenberg MS, Greenberg MS. Handbook of neurosurgery. Tampa (FL); New York: Greenberg Graphics; Thieme Medical Publishers; 2010.
11. Blumenfeld H. Neuroanatomy through clinical cases. Sunderland (MA): Sinauer; 2002.
12. Wilson-Pauwels L, Akesson EJ, Stewart PA. Cranial nerves: anatomy and clinical comments. Toronto; Philadelphia; St Louis (MO): BC Decker; CV Mosby; 1988 [distributor].
13. Olson DM, Stutzman SE, Saju C, et al. Interrater reliability of pupillary assessments. Neurocrit Care 2015. [Epub ahead of print].
14. Clark A, Clarke TN, Gregson B, et al. Variability in pupil size estimation. Emerg Med J 2006;23(6):440–1.
15. Litvan I, Saposnik G, Maurino J, et al. Pupillary diameter assessment: need for a graded scale. Neurology 2000;54(2):530–1.

16. Wilson SF, Amling JK, Floyd SD, et al. Determining interrater reliability of nurses' assessments of pupillary size and reaction. J Neurosci Nurs 1988;20(3):189–92.
17. Worthley LI. The pupillary light reflex in the critically ill patient. Crit Care Resusc 2000;2(1):7–8.
18. McMullen WH. The evolution of the ophthalmoscope. Br J Ophthalmol 1917;1: 593–9.
19. Hess EH, Polt JM. Pupil size as related to interest value of visual stimuli. Science 1960;132(3423):349–50.
20. Schallenberg M, Bangre V, Steuhl KP, et al. Comparison of the Colvard, Procyon, and Neuroptics pupillometers for measuring pupil diameter under low ambient illumination. J Refract Surg (Thorofare, NJ: 1995) 2010;26(2):134–43.
21. Chen JW, Vakil-Gilani K, Williamson KL, et al. Infrared pupillometry, the Neurological Pupil Index and unilateral pupillary dilation after traumatic brain injury: implications for treatment paradigms. Springerplus 2014;3:548.
22. Chen JW, Gombart ZJ, Rogers S, et al. Pupillary reactivity as an early indicator of increased intracranial pressure: the introduction of the Neurological Pupil Index. Surg Neurol Int 2011;2:82.
23. Song Z, Zheng W, Zhu H, et al. Prediction of coma and anisocoria based on computerized tomography findings in patients with supratentorial intracerebral hemorrhage. Clin Neurol Neurosurg 2012;114(6):634–8.
24. Greenberg MS, Arredondo N. Handbook of neurosurgery. 6th edition. Lakeland (FL); New York: Greenberg Graphics; Thieme Medical Publishers; 2006.
25. Braakman R, Gelpke GJ, Habbema JD, et al. Systematic selection of prognostic features in patients with severe head injury. Neurosurgery 1980;6(4):362–70.
26. Ritter AM, Muizelaar JP, Barnes T, et al. Brain stem blood flow, pupillary response, and outcome in patients with severe head injuries. Neurosurgery 1999;44(5): 941–8.
27. Meeker M, Du R, Bacchetti P, et al. Pupil examination: validity and clinical utility of an automated pupillometer. J Neurosci Nurs 2005;37(1):34–40.
28. Fountas KN, Kapsalaki EZ, Machinis TG, et al. Clinical implications of quantitative infrared pupillometry in neurosurgical patients. Neurocrit Care 2006;5(1):55–60.
29. Munoz Negrete FJ, Rebolleda G. Automated evaluation of the pupil. Arch Soc Esp Oftalmol 2013;88(4):125–6.
30. Du R, Meeker M, Bacchetti P, et al. Evaluation of the portable infrared pupillometer. Neurosurgery 2005;57(1):198–203 [discussion: 198–203].
31. Zafar SF, Suarez JI. Automated pupillometer for monitoring the critically ill patient: a critical appraisal. J Crit Care 2014;29(4):599–603.
32. Mahdavi Z, Pierre-Louis N, Ho T, et al. Advances in cerebral monitoring for the patient with traumatic brain injury. Crit Care Nurs Clin North Am 2015;27(2): 213–23.
33. Loewenfeld IE, Lowenstein O. The pupil: anatomy, physiology, and clinical applications. Ames (IL); Detroit (MI): Iowa State University Press; Wayne State University Press; 1993.
34. Goebert HW Jr. Head injury associated with a dilated pupil. Surg Clin North Am 1970;50(2):427–32.
35. Manley GT, Larson MD. Infrared pupillometry during uncal herniation. J Neurosurg Anesthesiol 2002;14(3):223–8.

Cerebral Microdialysis

Bethany Young, MSN, RN, AGCNS-BC[a],*, Atul Kalanuria, MD[b],
Monisha Kumar, MD[c], Kathryn Burke, BSN, RN[d], Ramani Balu, MD, PhD[b],
Olivia Amendolia, BA, BSN, RN[a], Kyle McNulty[a], BethAnn Marion, BSN, RN[a],
Brittany Beckmann, BSN, RN[a], Lauren Ciocco, BSN, RN[a], Kimberly Miller, BSN, RN[a],
Donnamarie Schuele, BSN, RN[a], Eileen Maloney-Wilensky, MSN, ACNP-BC[e],
Suzanne Frangos, RN, CNRN[e], Danielle Wright, BSN, RN[a]

KEYWORDS

- Cerebral microdialysis • Brain metabolism • Lactate/pyruvate ratio
- Brain energy crisis • Multimodality monitoring

KEY POINTS

- Cerebral microdialysis (CMD) provides a novel method of regional neuromonitoring of brain biochemistry at the cellular level.
- Controversy exists as to the optimal placement of the probe; however, most clinicians agree that placement in penumbral or perilesional tissue may have the most utility in guiding clinical interventions.
- CMD has been studied most rigorously in traumatic brain injury and subarachnoid hemorrhage, although it may be reasonable to use this monitor in any patient at risk for neurologic deterioration.
- The most commonly measured metabolites include glucose, lactate, pyruvate, glycerol, and glutamate; however, the number of analytes recovered and studied continues to grow.
- CMD is most often used in the treatment of severely injured neurocritical care patients as part of a multimodal approach that includes intracranial pressure monitoring, cerebral perfusion pressure monitoring, and brain tissue oxygen monitoring.

INTRODUCTION

The management of neurocritical care patients focuses on preservation of salvageable brain tissue and prevention of potentially avoidable secondary complications. Traditional neuromonitoring techniques include serial neurologic examination,

[a] Department of Nursing, Hospital of the University of Pennsylvania, 3400 Spruce Street, 2nd Floor Rhoads Building, Philadelphia, PA 19104, USA; [b] Department of Neurology, University of Pennsylvania, 3400 Spruce Street, 3 West Gates Building, Philadelphia, PA 19104, USA; [c] Department of Neurology, Perelman School of Medicine, University of Pennsylvania, 3400 Spruce Street, 3 West Gates Building, Philadelphia, PA 19104, USA; [d] Penn Presbyterian Medical Center, Philadelphia, PA 19104, USA; [e] Department of Neurosurgery, University of Pennsylvania, 3400 Spruce Street, 3 West Gates Building, Philadelphia, PA 19104, USA
* Corresponding author.
E-mail address: Bethany.young@uphs.upenn.edu

Crit Care Nurs Clin N Am 28 (2016) 109–124
http://dx.doi.org/10.1016/j.cnc.2015.09.005
0899-5885/16/$ – see front matter Published by Elsevier Inc.

ccnursing.theclinics.com

intracranial pressure (ICP) monitoring, brain tissue oxygenation ($P_{bt}O_2$) monitoring, serial imaging studies, and continuous electroencephalography. Despite clinical advances in the care of patients with severe brain injury, secondary ischemic and non-ischemic events remain a major cause of poor prognosis. Improved long-term patient outcomes depend on preemptive measures, early detection, and aggressive treatment of conditions that lead to secondary injury. Although basic monitors provide values that serve as proxies for brain health, they do not provide direct measurement of cerebral biochemistry, ischemia, or metabolism.

Cerebral microdialysis (CMD) allows bedside monitoring of the neurochemical state of the brain through collection and analysis of molecular substances from the brain's interstitial fluid. Molecules routinely recovered from brain interstitial fluid by CMD provide direct biochemical readouts of the level of cerebral ischemia (lactate, pyruvate), excitotoxicity (glutamate), and cell death (glycerol) in brain-injured patients that are not possible to obtain using conventional monitoring strategies. CMD has been used in laboratory settings and various clinical applications for several decades, although its use in humans was not initiated until 1992.[1,2] Levels and trends of the analytes obtained through CMD warn of impending detrimental secondary events in patients with severe neurologic compromise.[3,4] This article provides a guide to nursing personnel in the use of CMD and its nursing implications.

USEFULNESS AND INDICATIONS

The utility of CMD has been increasingly evident, with nearly 700 publications since its clinical debut.[5] CMD is indicated for use in patients with severe brain injury who are at risk for developing secondary cerebral hypoxia, ischemia, energy failure, and glucose deprivation and in whom the underlying neurologic status is unclear because of varying degrees of coma.[3,6] Variations in analyte levels reflect metabolic derangements (mainly deficient oxygen and/or glucose) that may signify mitochondrial failure, excitotoxic injury, or cell death within injured brain.[2,7] These changes may herald impending cerebral ischemia, epileptic activity, and intracranial hypertension.[7–12]

In combination with additional monitoring modalities, CMD may lend guidance to clinical decision making.[6–12] Results may guide systemic glucose management[13–20] and inform mean arterial pressure (MAP) and cerebral perfusion pressure (CPP) targets (**Fig. 1**)[21–25] as well as hemoglobin thresholds.[26] CMD may advise the safety and tolerability of episodic discontinuation of sedative infusions[27,28] and monitor cerebral metabolism after decompressive hemicraniectomy.[29,30] Furthermore, analysis of CMD analyte trends has shown correlation with long-term neurologic outcomes in both traumatic brain injury (TBI) and subarachnoid hemorrhage (SAH), which is useful in guiding prognostic efforts.[31–34]

Although CMD-guided algorithms have been most extensively studied in TBI and SAH, the physiologic data provided by CMD apply to brain injury from other causes, including intraparenchymal hemorrhage,[35] ischemic stroke,[36–38] brain tumors,[39] and hepatic encephalopathy.[40] In addition, it may be used to assess central nervous system penetration of pharmacologic agents, neurocytokines, and drug delivery, as well as serving as a biomarker or surrogate end point in research studies.[41,42]

CATHETER PLACEMENT

Cerebral microdialysis requires placement of a thin, fenestrated catheter into the subcortical white matter of the brain parenchyma. The catheter may be inserted through a single-lumen or multilumen cranial bolt system or tunneled percutaneously.

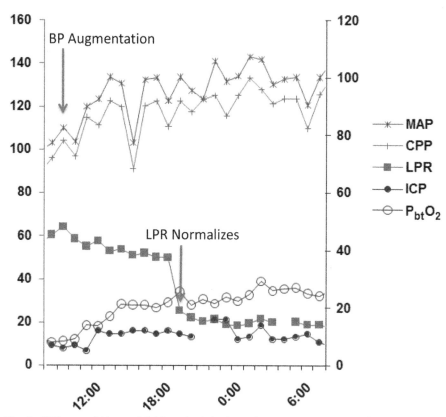

Fig. 1. CMD may aid in establishing physiologic goals to optimize MAP and CPP. This graph shows multimodality monitoring in a high-grade patient with subarachnoid hemorrhage (SAH) over a 24-hour period during the window of delayed cerebral ischemia. Initially, the lactate/pyruvate ratio (LPR) was increased, suggesting ischemia or cell energy crisis despite apparently normal MAP and CPP. ICP measurements at this time were below the traditional threshold for treatment. The patient's blood pressure (BP) was pharmacologically augmented to optimize MAP and CPP. Thereafter, the $P_{bt}O_2$ increased, and the LPR normalized. This finding shows the utility of CMD in guiding clinical treatment and corroborating results of other multimodality parameters to provide more granular detail than may be obtained from traditional monitoring devices.

Microdialysis monitors the local neurochemical environment contained within a radius of a few millimeters of the microdialysis catheter tip.[43] Therefore, precise positioning of the catheter is paramount to ensure that the collected data are consistent with the tissue region of interest.[4] Tunneling offers more accurate targeting of penumbral tissue, or tissue at risk.[42] However, tunneling the catheter is most often performed in the operating room, and may not be a viable option for those patients who do not require surgical intervention. Placement through a bolt may be performed in the intensive care unit, although this procedure is done with standard landmarks and without radiographic or fluoroscopic assistance. Placement through a bolt reduces the likelihood that the catheter will be directed at the penumbra or perilesional tissue.[42]

The appropriate location of probe may vary based on disease process. In patients with TBI, the catheter is typically placed into the pericontusional region of salvageable tissue. This tissue is known to be highly sensitive to perfusion varia-tions.[31] In patients with aneurysmal SAH, the catheter is placed in the region of the parent vessel at risk for vasospasm.[44,45] For disease states other than TBI or SAH, there are limited data to guide catheter placement. According to results of the Consensus Conference on Multimodality Monitoring in Neurocritical Care, loca-tion of the CMD probe should depend on the diagnosis, type, and location of the brain lesion, as well as the technical feasibility of placement.[6] Postinsertion, cath-eter placement is verified through visualization of the catheter tip by computed to-mography (CT).[44,46]

Timing and duration of probe placement should correspond with the period of high-est risk for secondary injury. For example, complications of TBI include formation of edema and derangements in cerebral blood flow and autoregulation, which tend to occur early in the treatment course. By contrast, in SAH, the major concern for secondary injury is vasospasm-associated ischemia, in which the onset and peak occurrence are delayed by days after hemorrhage. Timing of probe placement should allow for capture of baseline data.[41]

DEVICE AND TECHNIQUE

The monitoring device comprises a double-lumen dialysis probe that is inserted within brain tissue. After implantation, the catheter is connected to a battery-operated pump that continuously perfuses the brain with artificial cerebrospinal fluid or normal saline via the catheter at a rate of 0.3 μL/min per 10 mm of membrane length. The perfusion fluid is strategically isotonic to the brain interstitial fluid in order to permit the passive diffusion of small solutes from the interstitial fluid across the semipermeable portion of the cath-eter membrane and into the perfusion fluid. The perfusion fluid is then collected in small vials at hourly intervals. These vials are inserted into the analyzer and levels of certain small molecular substances are quantified (**Fig. 2**).[1] Note that these levels are not true absolute extracellular concentrations, but they reflect a relative recovery of the ana-lytes.[47] Flow rate, catheter length, and certain tissue properties influence mean relative recovery of substances. Tissue edema and tissue damage near the catheter membrane may reduce substance availability.[48] Fluctuations in ICP and protein concentration in the extracellular space may result in variable fluid recovery.[49]

The pore size of the catheter determines what size molecules may be taken up via CMD. There are commercially available 20-kD and 100-kD membrane probes, although only the smaller probes are US Food and Drug Administration approved in the United States at this time. The large 100-kD membrane probe is required for mea-surement of higher molecular weight molecules such as cytokines, inflammatory markers, some neurotransmitters, and certain medications.[50–52] Recovery of larger molecules may provide additional evidence that corroborates cautionary physiologic values and aids in prognostication.[52]

ANALYTES

The substances traditionally monitored with CMD are glucose, pyruvate, lactate, glutamate, and glycerol.[53] These values provide information about cellular metabolism (glucose, lactate, pyruvate), excitotoxicity (glutamate), and cell wall integrity (glycerol) (**Table 1**).[3]

Glucose

Glucose is the primary source of energy for the brain. Both high and low brain glucose levels are associated with unfavorable outcome, although an ideal

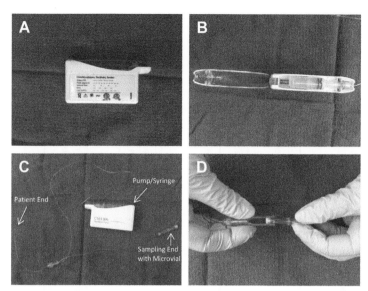

Fig. 2. (A) 106 Microdialysis pump. (B) 106 Microdialysis pump with syringe containing perfusion fluid. (C) 106 Microdialysis pump connected to 70 microdialysis bolt catheter. (D) Connecting microvial for dialysate collection. (*Courtesy of* (*A–D*), M Dialysis AB, Stockholm, Sweden; with permission.)

glucose range has not been determined.[13,22,31,32,54–56] Brain glucose concentration reflects serum glucose levels, although this relationship may be altered in the setting of brain injury.[13–18,57,58] Brain glucose levels may also change with alterations in brain capillary perfusion. Consideration of the relationship between changing brain glucose concentrations and systemic glucose concentration helps guide the decision to modify systemic glucose management or address deficiencies in brain capillary perfusion.[45,59] Systemic glucose level variability may precipitate cerebral metabolic distress and negatively affect patient outcome. Avoiding acute fluctuations in systemic glucose levels should be a goal of patient management.[22]

Pyruvate and Lactate

After glucose enters the cell, it is converted to pyruvate through the process of glycolysis. Under normal, aerobic conditions, pyruvate is converted to acetyl coenzyme A, which then enters the citric acid cycle to produce a net energy yield of 36 ATP. In a hypoxic state, pyruvate is unable to undergo aerobic metabolism and is therefore anaerobically metabolized to lactate. This process results in a much lower energy yield of only 2 ATP.[2,60]

Lactate and pyruvate both freely diffuse across the cell membrane, making intracellular accumulation of lactate and depletion of pyruvate apparent in the extracellular fluid (ECF) and detectable by CMD.[53] Because lactate and pyruvate levels can be affected by multiple factors, the lactate/pyruvate ratio (LPR) is a more specific marker of ischemia than either marker is in isolation.[60] Increased LPR is traditionally interpreted to signify cerebral ischemia; however, LPR can be increased in both ischemic and nonischemic states.[2] An increased LPR with low oxygen and low pyruvate levels indicates ischemia.[5] Increased LPR with normal oxygen and normal to high pyruvate levels can indicate mitochondrial dysfunction (energy failure),[5,61] but also may also represent a normal variant,

Table 1
CMD analytes and clinical application

Analyte	Normal Value[a]	Pathologic Threshold	Clinical Significance	Outcome Relationship
Glucose	1.5–2 mM	<0.2 mM	Primary energy source for the brain. Derangements in cerebral glucose levels may result from ischemia, hyperemia, hyperglycemia/hypoglycemia, or hypermetabolism/hypometabolism	Unfavorable outcomes associated with both low and high cerebral glucose levels
Lactate	3 mmol/L	>4 mmol/L	Substrate of anaerobic metabolism. Not a reliable marker in isolation	Increases with hypoxia/ischemia
Pyruvate	120 μM	Not defined	Enters citric acid cycle for energy production under aerobic conditions or is converted to lactate under anaerobic conditions. Interpreted in conjunction with lactate, $P_{bt}O_2$, and glucose levels. Not a reliable marker in isolation	Decreases with hypoxia/ischemia
LPR	15–20	>25	Very sensitive to ischemic and hypoxic changes	Increased LPR is associated with unfavorable outcome
Glutamate	10 μM	Not defined	Excitatory amino acid and neurotransmitter. Excess in the extracellular space results from excessive release or impaired cellular uptake. Early, indirect marker of cellular damage and failing energy levels	Prolonged, increased levels thought to be an additional injurious mechanism and may exacerbate injury in TBI and SAH
Glycerol	50–100 μM	Not defined	Indicator of cell membrane breakdown. Potential causes of increasing levels include cellular stress, hypoxia, and low glucose levels	No definitive evidence of a relationship between glycerol and patient outcome

Abbreviation: LPR, lactate/pyruvate ratio.
[a] Normal values based on a 20-kD dialysis membrane, 10 mm in length, and perfusion flow of 0.3 μL/min.

because neurons can use lactate produced by astrocytes for oxidative metabolism (especially during increases in brain activity).[62] Differentiating the causes of increased LPR may determine treatment pathways.[61] Increased LPR is consistently associated with unfavorable outcomes across a variety of diagnoses.[22,31,32,34,35,54,63–68]

Glutamate

Glutamate is an excitatory neurotransmitter and amino acid in the central nervous system. Significant increases in extracellular glutamate levels have been observed following central nervous system injury.[5,69] Excess of extracellular excitatory amino acids leads to receptor overactivation; interruption of ion homeostasis; and subsequent neuronal injury, including acute neuronal swelling, cell membrane degradation, and cellular death.[33,69–71] Increases in extracellular glutamate levels have been observed in the setting of ischemia[5,37,59,72,73] and epileptiform activity.[73–76]

Measuring cerebral glutamate by microdialysis is an option and may be useful for prognostication and clinical guidance. In patients with TBI, increased glutamate levels, particularly those that progressively increase over time or remain significantly increased, may be predictive of poor patient outcome and worse 6-month functional outcome than those of patients whose glutamate levels normalize over time.[33] Profound increases in glutamate levels have also been observed in patients with SAH in the setting of cerebral ischemia before the onset of symptomatic vasospasm.[5,10,11] Prolonged increased glutamate levels may also indicate impending increased ICP.[30]

Glycerol

Glycerol is an integral component of the cell membrane; thus, increased glycerol concentrations in interstitial fluid indicate cell membrane decomposition and cell death. When oxygen and glucose delivery is deficient, as in the setting of ischemia, calcium transporters that actively shuttle calcium out of the cell are not activated, allowing calcium to leak into the cell. This leakage activates phospholipases, which in turn break down the cell membrane and release glycerol into the ECF.[1] Increased cerebral glycerol may serve as a marker of cerebral injury; however, its specificity is limited and levels are influenced by systemic concentrations. Further investigation is needed to determine a definitive relationship between glycerol and outcome.[5]

DATA INTERPRETATION

A simple approach to interpreting CMD data is to remember the LTC (level, trend, and comparison) method.[45] First, are the results within or outside the normal range? Second, are the results becoming more or less pathologic over time? Trends of CMD analytes are equally if not more important than stand-alone values or strict threshold values.[5] Third, how do the results compare with values and trends of other physiologic parameters?[45]

Recommendations from the 2014 International Microdialysis Forum and a body of accumulating evidence suggest consideration of CMD analytes in a tiered hierarchy (**Box 1**).

- Tier 1: glucose and LPR
- Tier 2: glutamate
- Tier 3: glycerol

Tier 1 is considered the most robust for clinical use based on quantity of data supporting greater outcomes and greater potential to directly affect clinical intervention.[5]

Box 1
Tiered approach to interpretation of CMD data and interventions

Increased lactate level or LPR GREATER THAN 25

If lactate level or LPR are increased without a decrease in cerebral glucose level (<0.7) or decrease in $P_{bt}O_2$ consider watchful waiting.

Assess and treat causes of increased lactate level:

- Inadequate O_2 delivery/cerebral ischemia
  - Systemic hypotension/shock: evaluate and treat accordingly
  - Systemic hypoxia: optimize pulmonary function, goal partial pressure arterial oxygen greater than 100
  - Anemia: consider red blood cell transfusion if hemoglobin level less than 9
  - New structural lesion (hemorrhage or stroke) consider imaging with CT or MRI
  - Delayed ischemic neurologic deficit or vasospasm: consider trial of induced hypertension and/or vascular imaging
- Cerebral metabolic crisis (LPR >25 and glucose level <0.7, with normal $P_{bt}O_2$ and ICP); consider trial of induced hypertension to augment CPP
- Increased brain O_2 demand
  - Fever: treat accordingly; if prolonged, consider targeted temperature management
  - Seizures: consider electroencephalogram (EEG) monitoring
  - Shivering/rigors: consider trial of neuromuscular blockade
- Abnormal systemic lactate clearance/production
  - Acute liver failure
  - Sepsis (leads to catecholamine-induced beta-receptor stimulation): can occur without hypotension
- Uncoupling of oxidative phosphorylation (medications/toxins)
  - Propofol
  - Lorazepam
  - Cyanide
  - Carbon monoxide
  - Toxic ingestions (eg, methanol, ethylene glycol)

Consider trial of induced hypertension to increase CPP if work-up unrevealing.

Increased glutamate level

Assess causes of increased glutamate level:

- Seizures: consider EEG monitoring
- New acute structural lesion (especially infarction): consider imaging with CT or MRI
- Excitotoxicity: consider imaging with CT or MRI
- Acute liver failure

Increased glycerol level

Increases in glycerol level suggest acute cellular necrosis.

- New acute structural lesion (hemorrhage, infarct): consider imaging with CT or MRI

CMD data are most meaningful when interpreted in relation to other data points, such as ICP, CPP, $P_{bt}O_2$, and cerebral blood flow.[45] It is extremely difficult to draw associations between data points when the data are presented in table format. Linear graphs that time match data from multiple monitors allow much clearer correlation of data points. A component neuromonitoring system may aid in clinical decision making with CMD because it integrates physiologic data from all patient devices into a graphical format on a single monitor.

SAFETY PROFILE

CMD catheter placement is generally a safe practice. As with the placement of any intracerebral monitoring device, safety concerns in relation to CMD catheter placement include hemorrhage, infection, and catheter dislodgment. Multiple published studies have reported the safety of CMD catheter insertion, including a study by Chen and colleagues[39] in which no hemorrhage or infection was attributable to CMD out of a sample of 174 patients.[5,10,77–79] The safety profile of CMD is comparable with, and may be greater than, that of intraparenchymal pressure sensors owing to the CMD catheter's relative flexibility and small diameter.[80]

PREPARATION FOR CLINICAL APPLICATION

Preparing for use of CMD in a clinical setting requires fastidious planning and extensive multidisciplinary collaboration (**Box 2**). It is essential to initiate early and frequent communication between key stakeholders to ensure cohesive expectations and to prevent delays in clinical implementation (**Table 2**). The objective for using CMD should be transparent to all parties, meaning whether it is intended for use as a standard to guide clinical care, as a research mechanism, or a combination of both. This decision helps to determine priority stakeholders and ownership of the process while always maintaining the priority of the patient.

NURSING CONSIDERATIONS

Nursing plays an integral role in successfully implementing CMD at the bedside. The nurse is responsible for assisting the provider during insertion of the catheter, collecting hourly samples, operating the analyzer, documenting laboratory results, communicating results to the appropriate provider, maintaining the catheter and pump, and conducting ongoing family education. Samples are routinely collected every 60 minutes or potentially at shorter intervals (as frequently as every 10 minutes) if clinically indicated. Throughout the duration of CMD, the nurse

---

Box 2
Implementation of CMD in a clinical setting is a multidisciplinary effort reaching far beyond bedside personnel. Communication between representatives from each of the listed groups should be coordinated at regular intervals to ensure buy-in from key stakeholders

Neurocritical care faculty and trainees

Neurocritical care nurses

Neurosurgery attendings and residents

Point of care personnel

Information technology

Research division

Hospital products and purchasing department

CMD vendor

Table 2
Clinical application of CMD requires coordination and consideration of many factors involving multiple disciplines

Consideration	Action
Protocol development	Combined multidisciplinary creation/ratification of pathway/algorithm to guide clinical care
Nursing staffing	1:1 assignment
Physical setup	Analyzer centrally located on unit Access to network Ethernet Access to supplies
Training	Catheter insertion: neurosurgery Medical management: neurocritical care Physical care/monitoring/analyzer operations: nursing Analyzer maintenance and operations: point-of-care personnel
Documentation	Electronic vs paper
Supply approval and purchasing	Collaborate with purchasing and supply personnel
Downtime plan	Plan for refrigerated storage of samples to be run after analyzer function is restored
Data storage	Liaise with hospital information technology department
Interface with other neuromonitoring parameters	Consider component neuromonitoring system
Research implications	Consider research opportunities to be performed simultaneously with clinical care

---

monitors for any fluid leakage or signs of infection at the catheter insertion site, and monitors the pump for active battery life.[3] Because of the intensity of nursing care associated with CMD, patients requiring microdialysis should be 1:1 nursing assignments.

The method and location for documentation of CMD results are critical to successful implementation. Hourly results may be printed from the CMD analyzer; however, institutional capability of directly transferring results into the electronic medical record (EMR) is done in collaboration with the hospital's information technology department. The nurse is likely to need to manually transcribe CMD data into the EMR or onto a customized paper flow sheet (**Fig. 3**). It is advisable to document CMD values in a format or location in which the trends can easily be compared with other neuromonitoring parameters. Clinical events and medical interventions should be documented on the CMD data collection sheet. This practice allows for observation of the relationship between clinical findings or targeted interventions with CMD values.

Formulation of a plan in the event of an operational downtime is necessary to ensure seamless ongoing collection and preservation of patient samples. Samples may be refrigerated for several days because preservation and stability of samples increases at lower temperatures.

Limited amounts of patient data may be temporarily stored in the analyzer; however, long-term storage of results requires transfer to an external source. Liaising with the hospital information technology department can be instrumental in identifying sufficient protected space for storage of large quantities of patient-sensitive data.

Place pt label here.

DATE:

Exam Change:

Intervention:

	0700	0800	0900	1000	1100	1200	1300	1400	1500	1600	1700	1800
ICP												
CPP												
$P_{bt}O_2$												
Brain temperature												
CBF												
K Value												
Microdialysis Values:												
Glucose												
Lactate												
Pyruvate												
LPR												
Glutamate												
Glycerol												

Fig. 3. Example of an MMM (multimodality monitoring) nursing documentation grid depicting hour CMD analyte values alongside other neuromonitoring parameters.

SUMMARY

Sequelae of secondary brain injury following TBI or SAH are leading contributors to poor prognoses. The goals of neurocritical care are to prevent the onset and extent of damage from secondary injury. In order to achieve these goals, more information is often needed than can be obtained from traditional neuromonitoring techniques. CMD is a bedside clinical tool that provides information regarding localized cerebral cellular metabolism, excitotoxicity, and cell wall integrity.[3] Practical implementation of CMD for clinical use requires multidisciplinary engagement in order to ensure adequate training and education, preparation of the physical environment, regulatory compliance, and meaningful protocol development. In conjunction with data from other devices, CMD may inform clinical decision making, guide medical interventions, and aid in prognostication efforts.[6]

REFERENCES

1. Kitagawa R, Yokobori S, Mazzeo AT, et al. Microdialysis in the neurocritical care unit. Neurosurg Clin North Am 2013;24(3):417–26.
2. Larach DB, Kofke WA, Le Roux P. Potential non-hypoxic/ischemic causes of increased cerebral interstitial fluid lactate/pyruvate ratio: a review of available literature. Neurocrit Care 2011;15(3):609–22.
3. Presciutti M, Schmidt JM, Alexander S. Neuromonitoring in intensive care: focus on microdialysis and its nursing implications. J Neurosci Nurs 2009;41(3):131–9.
4. De Lima Oliveira M, Kairalla AC, Fonoff ET, et al. Cerebral microdialysis in traumatic brain injury and subarachnoid hemorrhage: state of the art. Neurocrit Care 2014;21(1):152–62.
5. Hutchinson PJ, Jalloh I, Helmy A, et al. Consensus statement from the 2014 international microdialysis forum. Intensive Care Med 2015;41(9):1517–28.
6. Le Roux P, Menon DK, Citerio G, et al. Consensus summary statement of the International Multidisciplinary Consensus Conference on Multimodality Monitoring in Neurocritical Care: a statement for healthcare professionals from the Neurocritical Care Society and the European Society of Intensive Care Medicine. Intensive Care Med 2014;40(9):1189–209.
7. Belli A, Sen J, Petzold A, et al. Metabolic failure precedes intracranial pressure rises in traumatic brain injury: a microdialysis study. Acta Neurochir (Wien) 2008;150(5):461–9.
8. Adamides AA, Rosenfeldt FL, Winter CD, et al. Brain tissue lactate elevations predict episodes of intracranial hypertension in patients with traumatic brain injury. J Am Coll Surg 2009;209(4):531–9.
9. Skjøth-Rasmussen J, Schulz M, Kristensen SR, et al. Delayed neurological deficits detected by an ischemic pattern in the extracellular cerebral metabolites in patients with aneurysmal subarachnoid hemorrhage. J Neurosurg 2004;100(1):8–15.
10. Sarrafzadeh AS, Sakowitz OW, Kiening KL, et al. Bedside microdialysis: a tool to monitor cerebral metabolism in subarachnoid hemorrhage patients? Crit Care Med 2002;30(5):1062–70.
11. Unterberg AW, Sakowitz OW, Sarrafzadeh AS, et al. Role of bedside microdialysis in the diagnosis of cerebral vasospasm following aneurysmal subarachnoid hemorrhage. J Neurosurg 2001;94:740–9.
12. Nilsson OG, Brandt L, Ungerstedt U, et al. Bedside detection of brain ischemia using intracerebral microdialysis: subarachnoid hemorrhage and delayed ischemic deterioration. Neurosurgery 1999;45(5):1176–85.

13. Oddo M, Schmidt JM, Carrera E, et al. Impact of tight glycemic control on cerebral glucose metabolism after severe brain injury: a microdialysis study. Crit Care Med 2008;36(12):3233–8.
14. Vespa P, McArthur DL, Stein N, et al. Tight glycemic control increases metabolic distress in traumatic brain injury. Crit Care Med 2012;40(6):1923–9.
15. Vespa P, Boonyaputthikul R, McArthur DL, et al. Intensive insulin therapy reduces microdialysis glucose values without altering glucose utilization or improving the lactate/pyruvate ratio after traumatic brain injury. Crit Care Med 2006;34(3): 850–6.
16. Zetterling M, Hillered L, Enblad P, et al. Relation between brain interstitial and systemic glucose concentrations after subarachnoid hemorrhage. J Neurosurg 2011;115(1):66–74.
17. Magnoni S, Tedesco C, Carbonara M, et al. Relationship between systemic glucose and cerebral glucose is preserved in patients with severe traumatic brain injury, but glucose delivery to the brain may become limited when oxidative metabolism is impaired. Crit Care Med 2012;40(6):1785–91.
18. Rostami E, Bellander B-M. Monitoring of glucose in brain, adipose tissue, and peripheral blood in patients with traumatic brain injury: a microdialysis study. J Diabetes Sci Technol 2011;5(3):596–604. Available at: http://www.pubmedcentral.nih.gov/articlerender.fcgi?artid=3192626&tool=pmcentrez&rendertype=abstract.
19. Schlenk F, Nagel A, Graetz D. Hyperglycemia and cerebral glucose in aneurysmal subarachnoid hemorrhage. Intensive Care Med 2008;34(7):1200–7.
20. Helbok R, Schmidt JM, Kurtz P, et al. Systemic glucose and brain energy metabolism after subarachnoid hemorrhage. Neurocrit Care 2010;12(3):317–23.
21. Nordström C-H, Reinstrup P, Xu W, et al. Assessment of the lower limit for cerebral perfusion pressure in severe head injuries by bedside monitoring of regional energy metabolism. Anesthesiology 2003;98(4):809–14.
22. Schmidt JM, Ko SB, Helbok R, et al. Cerebral perfusion pressure thresholds for brain tissue hypoxia and metabolic crisis after poor-grade subarachnoid hemorrhage. Stroke 2011;42(5):1351–6.
23. Johnston AJ, Steiner LA, Coles JP, et al. Effect of cerebral perfusion pressure augmentation on regional oxygenation and metabolism after head injury. Crit Care Med 2005;33(1):189–95 [discussion: 255–7].
24. Johnston AJ, Steiner LA, Chatfield DA, et al. Effect of cerebral perfusion pressure augmentation with dopamine and norepinephrine on global and focal brain oxygenation after traumatic brain injury. Intensive Care Med 2004;30(5):791–7.
25. Chen HI, Stiefel MF, Oddo M, et al. Detection of cerebral compromise with multimodality monitoring in patients with subarachnoid hemorrhage. Neurosurgery 2011;69(1):53–63.
26. Oddo M, Milby A, Chen I, et al. Hemoglobin concentration and cerebral metabolism in patients with aneurysmal subarachnoid hemorrhage. Stroke 2009; 40(4):1275–81.
27. Helbok R, Kurtz P, Schmidt MJ, et al. Effects of the neurological wake-up test on clinical examination, intracranial pressure, brain metabolism and brain tissue oxygenation in severely brain-injured patients. Crit Care 2012;16(6):R226.
28. Skoglund K, Hillered L, Purins K, et al. The neurological wake-up test does not alter cerebral energy metabolism and oxygenation in patients with severe traumatic brain injury. Neurocrit Care 2014;20(3):413–26.
29. Ho CL, Wang CM, Lee KK, et al. Cerebral oxygenation, vascular reactivity, and neurochemistry following decompressive craniectomy for severe traumatic brain injury. J Neurosurg 2008;108(5):943–9.

30. Nagel A, Graetz D, Vajkoczy P, et al. Decompressive craniectomy in aneurysmal subarachnoid hemorrhage: relation to cerebral perfusion pressure and metabolism. Neurocrit Care 2009;11(3):384–94.
31. Timofeev I, Carpenter KLH, Nortje J, et al. Cerebral extracellular chemistry and outcome following traumatic brain injury: a microdialysis study of 223 patients. Brain 2011;134(2):484–94.
32. Stein NR, McArthur DL, Etchepare M, et al. Early cerebral metabolic crisis after TBI influences outcome despite adequate hemodynamic resuscitation. Neurocrit Care 2012;17(1):49–57.
33. Chamoun R, Suki D, Gopinath SP, et al. Role of extracellular glutamate measured by cerebral microdialysis in severe traumatic brain injury. J Neurosurg 2010; 113(3):564–70.
34. Marcoux J, McArthur DA, Miller C, et al. Persistent metabolic crisis as measured by elevated cerebral microdialysis lactate-pyruvate ratio predicts chronic frontal lobe brain atrophy after traumatic brain injury. Crit Care Med 2008;36(10):2871–7.
35. Nikaina I, Paterakis K, Paraforos G, et al. Cerebral perfusion pressure, microdialysis biochemistry, and clinical outcome in patients with spontaneous intracerebral hematomas. J Crit Care 2012;27(1):83–8.
36. Berger C, Schäbitz WR, Georgiadis D, et al. Effects of hypothermia on excitatory amino acids and metabolism in stroke patients: a microdialysis study. Stroke 2002;33(2):519–24.
37. Dohmen C, Bosche B, Graf R, et al. Prediction of malignant course in MCA infarction by PET and microdialysis. Stroke 2003;34(9):2152–8.
38. Schneweis S, Grond M, Staub F, et al. Predictive value of neurochemical monitoring in large middle cerebral artery infarction. Stroke 2001;32(8):1863–7.
39. Chen J, Gombart Z, Cecil S, et al. Implementation of cerebral microdialysis at a community-based hospital: a 5-year retrospective analysis. Surg Neurol Int 2012; 3(1):57.
40. Tofteng F, Jorgensen L, Adel Hansen B, et al. Cerebral microdialysis in patients with fulminant hepatic failure. Hepatology 2002;36(6):1333–40.
41. Miller CM. Cerebral microdialysis. In: Torbey MT, Miller CM, editors. Neurocritical care monitoring, vol.. New York: Demos Medical Publishing; 2015. p. 70–84.
42. Frontera J, Ziai W, O'Phelan K, et al. Regional brain monitoring in the neurocritical care unit. Neurocrit Care 2015;22(3):348–59.
43. Engström M, Polito A, Reinstrup P, et al. Intracerebral microdialysis in severe brain trauma: the importance of catheter location. J Neurosurg 2005;102(3):460–9.
44. Cecil S, Chen PM, Callaway SE, et al. Traumatic brain injury advanced multimodal neuromonitoring from theory to clinical practice. Crit Care Nurse 2011;31(2): 25–37.
45. Ungerstedt U, Rostami E. Microdialysis in neurointensive care. Curr Pharm Des 2004;10(18):2145–52.
46. Ståhl N, Schalén W, Ungerstedt U, et al. Bedside biochemical monitoring of the penumbra zone surrounding an evacuated acute subdural haematoma. Acta Neurol Scand 2003;108:211–5.
47. Borg A, Smith M. Cerebral microdialysis: research technique or clinical tool? NeuroMethods 2013;75:1–21.
48. Hutchinson PJ, O'Connell MT, Al-Rawi PG, et al. Clinical cerebral microdialysis: a methodological study. J Neurosurg 2000;93(1):37–43.
49. Helmy A, Carpenter KLH, Menon DK, et al. The cytokine response to human traumatic brain injury: temporal profiles and evidence for cerebral parenchymal production. J Cereb Blood Flow Metab 2011;31(2):658–70.

50. Helmy A, Carpenter KLH, Skepper JN, et al. Microdialysis of cytokines: methodological considerations, scanning electron microscopy, and determination of relative recovery. J Neurotrauma 2009;26(4):549–61.
51. Hutchinson PJ, O'Connell MT, Nortje J, et al. Cerebral microdialysis methodology–evaluation of 20 kDa and 100 kDa catheters. Physiol Meas 2005;26(4):423–8.
52. Petzold A, Tisdall MM, Girbes AR, et al. In vivo monitoring of neuronal loss in traumatic brain injury: a microdialysis study. Brain 2011;134(2):464–83.
53. Goodman JC, Robertson CS. Microdialysis: is it ready for prime time? Curr Opin Crit Care 2009;15(2):110–7.
54. Dizdarevic K, Hamdan A, Omerhodzic I, et al. Modified Lund concept versus cerebral perfusion pressure-targeted therapy: a randomised controlled study in patients with secondary brain ischaemia. Clin Neurol Neurosurg 2012;114(2):142–8.
55. Vespa PM, McArthur D, O'Phelan K, et al. Persistently low extracellular glucose correlates with poor outcome 6 months after human traumatic brain injury despite a lack of increased lactate: a microdialysis study. J Cereb Blood Flow Metab 2003;23(7):865–77.
56. Cesarini KG, Enblad P, Ronne-Engström E, et al. Early cerebral hyperglycolysis after subarachnoid haemorrhage correlates with favourable outcome. Acta Neurochir (Wien) 2002;144(11):1121–31.
57. Schlenk F, Graetz D, Nagel A, et al. Insulin-related decrease in cerebral glucose despite normoglycemia in aneurysmal subarachnoid hemorrhage. Crit Care 2008;12(1):R9.
58. Schmidt JM, Claassen J, Ko S-B, et al. Nutritional support and brain tissue glucose metabolism in poor-grade SAH: a retrospective observational study. Crit Care 2012;16(1):R15.
59. Hlatky R, Valadka AB, Goodman JC, et al. Patterns of energy substrates during ischemia measured in the brain by microdialysis. J Neurotrauma 2004;21(7):894–906.
60. Johnston AJ, Gupta AK. Advanced monitoring in the neurology intensive care unit: microdialysis. Curr Opin Crit Care 2002;8(2):121–7.
61. Nielsen TH, Olsen NV, Toft P, et al. Cerebral energy metabolism during mitochondrial dysfunction induced by cyanide in piglets. Acta Anaesthesiol Scand 2013;57(6):793–801.
62. Oddo M, Levine JM, Frangos S, et al. Brain lactate metabolism in humans with subarachnoid hemorrhage. Stroke 2012;43(5):1418–21.
63. Sarrafzadeh A, Haux D, Küchler I, et al. Poor-grade aneurysmal subarachnoid hemorrhage: relationship of cerebral metabolism to outcome. J Neurosurg 2004;100(3):400–6.
64. Paraforou T, Paterakis K, Fountas K, et al. Cerebral perfusion pressure, microdialysis biochemistry and clinical outcome in patients with traumatic brain injury. BMC Res Notes 2011;4(1):540.
65. Samuelsson C, Hillered L, Enblad P, et al. Microdialysis patterns in subarachnoid hemorrhage patients with focus on ischemic events and brain interstitial glutamine levels. Acta Neurochir (Wien) 2009;151(5):437–46.
66. Vespa PM, Miller C, McArthur D, et al. Nonconvulsive electrographic seizures after traumatic brain injury result in a delayed, prolonged increase in intracranial pressure and metabolic crisis. Crit Care Med 2007;35(12):2830–6.
67. Kett-White R, Hutchinson PJ, Al-Rawi PG, et al. Adverse cerebral events detected after subarachnoid hemorrhage using brain oxygen and microdialysis probes. Neurosurgery 2002;50(6):1213–22.

68. Reinstrup P, Ståhl N, Mellergård P, et al. Intracerebral microdialysis in clinical practice: baseline values for chemical markers during wakefulness, anesthesia, and neurosurgery. Neurosurgery 2000;47(3):701–10.
69. Gentile NT, McIntosh TK. Antagonists of excitatory amino acids and endogenous opioid peptides in the treatment of experimental central nervous system injury. Ann Emerg Med 1993;22(6):1028–34.
70. Foster AC, Fagg GE. Neurobiology. Taking apart NMDA receptors. Nature 1987; 329(6138):395–6.
71. Cifuentes Castro VH, Lopez Valenzuela CL, Salazar Sanchez JC, et al. An update of the classical and novel methods used for measuring fast neurotransmitters during normal and brain altered function. Curr Neuropharmacol 2014;12(6):490–508.
72. Enblad P, Valtysson J, Andersson J, et al. Simultaneous intracerebral microdialysis and positron emission tomography in the detection of ischemia in patients with subarachnoid hemorrhage. J Cereb Blood Flow Metab 1996;16:637–44.
73. Vespa P, Prins M, Ronne-Engstrom E, et al. Increase in extracellular glutamate caused by reduced cerebral perfusion pressure and seizures after human traumatic brain injury: a microdialysis study. J Neurosurg 1998;89(6):971–82.
74. During MJ, Spencer DD. Extracellular hippocampal glutamate and spontaneous seizure in the conscious human brain. Lancet 1993;341(8861):1607–10.
75. Ronne-Engström E, Hillered L, Flink R, et al. Intracerebral microdialysis of extracellular amino acids in the human epileptic focus. J Cereb Blood Flow Metab 1992;12(5):873–6.
76. Kinoshita K, Moriya T, Utagawa A, et al. Change in brain glucose after enteral nutrition in subarachnoid hemorrhage. J Surg Res 2010;162(2):221–4.
77. Agren-Wilsson A, Roslin M, Eklund A, et al. Intracerebral microdialysis and CSF hydrodynamics in idiopathic adult hydrocephalus syndrome. J Neurol Neurosurg Psychiatry 2003;74(2):217–21.
78. Eide PK, Stanisic M. Cerebral microdialysis and intracranial pressure monitoring in patients with idiopathic normal-pressure hydrocephalus: association with clinical response to extended lumbar drainage and shunt surgery. J Neurosurg 2010; 112(2):414–24.
79. Zauner A, Doppenberg EMR, Woodward JJ, et al. Continuous monitoring of cerebral substrate delivery and clearance: initial experience in 24 patients with severe acute brain injuries. Neurosurgery 1997;41(5):1082–93.
80. Stuart RM, Schmidt M, Kurtz P, et al. Intracranial multimodal monitoring for acute brain injury: a single institution review of current practices. Neurocrit Care 2010; 12(2):188–98.

Targeted Temperature Modulation in the Neuroscience Patient

Marie Wilson, MSN, RN, CRNP, CCRN, CNRN*,
Amy Della Penna, MSN, RN, CCRN

KEYWORDS

- Targeted temperature management • Induced hypothermia • Normothermia
- Shivering

KEY POINTS

- Both induced hypothermia and normothermia means of improving outcomes in neurologically challenged patients have been a continued topic of discussion in the critical care literature.
- The need for a collaborative approach to best facilitate targeted temperature management (TTM) strategies and to minimize potential complications is warranted.
- Evidence-based standardized protocols are lacking; thus, initiation of treatment might be delayed by nurses' knowledge of fever management as well as individual physician orders.

INTRODUCTION

The American Heart Association's supported practice of therapeutic hypothermia (32°C–34°C for 12–24 hours) in out-of-hospital adult post–cardiac arrest comatose patients, as well as research on controlled hypothermia for neonates with hypoxic/ischemic encephalopathy, provides for key positioning in improving neurologic outcomes based on controlling temperature postinsult.[1,2] Based on the premise that brain cells die due to complex biochemical processes and postinflammatory cascade, utilization of TTM protocols, both induced hypothermia (32°C–34°C) and controlled normothermia (36°C–37°C),[3] as a means of improving outcomes in neurologically challenged patients has been a continued topic of discussion.

Disclosure Statement: The authors have nothing to disclose.
Neuroscience Intensive Care Unit, Thomas Jefferson University Hospital, 111 South 11th Street, Gibbon Building, Room 9300, Philadelphia, PA 19107, USA
* Corresponding author.
E-mail address: Marie.Wilson@jefferson.edu

Crit Care Nurs Clin N Am 28 (2016) 125–136
http://dx.doi.org/10.1016/j.cnc.2015.10.006
0899-5885/16/$ – see front matter
ccnursing.theclinics.com

FEVER

Fever is a normal cytokine-mediated immunologic reaction to infection or inflammation; however, hyperthermia in brain-injured patients can also be as the result of dysregulation within the hypothalamus aberrantly shifting the set point, which can also lead to secondary brain injury.[4,5] Healthy adult brains have the ability to tolerate fluctuations in temperature; however, the same variations in temperatures in compromised brains have been shown to increase ischemia and injury.[6]

There are 3 major reasons for elevated temperature in critically ill patients: infectious fever, noninfectious fever (including neurogenic fever, thrombophlebotic events, transfusion reactions, and drug fevers), and hyperthermic events (including malignant hyperthermia), with identification of a majority of fevers in patients with brain injury attributable to a pulmonary source.[4] In 1 of 5 to 1 of 3 of cases, the cause of fever remains unexplained despite aggressive work-up, leading to a belief that the cause may be central in origin.[7]

The underlying mechanism of these phenomena is thought due to several coexisting processes. Acute stress situations (such as response to injury), which in turn elevate body temperature, lead to stimulation of the autonomic centers within the right insular cortex, amygdala, and hypothalamus, which increases sympathetic outflow.[8] This heightened sympathetic response leads to increased heart rate, minute ventilation, oxygen consumption, and resting energy consumption. This concept can also be linked to increasing cerebral metabolic demand, which further stresses the injured brain, predisposing it to secondary injury. It has been hypothesized that for each 1°C increase in core body temperature, a corresponding 7% to 13% increase in cerebral metabolism may be experienced.[9] This increased metabolic demand at the cellular level coupled with diminished blood flow from injury further exacerbates the situation.[6] Fever is also known to increase the inflammatory process, which compromises the blood-brain barrier, leading to cerebral edema and neuronal death, as well as increasing production of free radicals due to excessive catecholamine release, inducing calcium influx and prolonged cellular excitation as a result of glutamate release.[10]

On a fundamental level, much debate has surrounded defining temperature measurement methodology. Normothermia has been described as 37°C, factoring in diurnal variations up to 1°C and acknowledging that axillary and oral temperatures are slightly less than core temperature but more easily obtainable than rectal, bladder, esophageal, or pulmonary artery catheter temperatures.[10,11] Definitions of "fever" include temperatures varying between 37.1°C and 38.5°C, with many suggesting intervention for any temperature greater than 37.5°C,[5] noting the importance of acknowledging that brain temperature is often higher than core body temperature and, as patients experience a febrile condition, the disparity between brain and core body temperatures increases.[12] This leads to belief that the diagnosis of fever in neurologically impaired populations may be underestimated and the treatment underused.

Neuroscience critical care research has suggested that after controlling for diagnosis, severity of illness, age, and complications, elevation in body temperature consistently can be linked to longer length of stay, higher mortality, and worse economic and functional outcomes.[13] Controlling fever can lead toward establishment of normal body physiology and lead toward a goal of recovery.

HISTORICAL PERSPECTIVE

The history of cooling patients for medical treatment was initiated by several early clinicians. In 1766, John Hunter, a physiologist, investigated animals exposed to extreme subnormal temperatures and then rewarmed having successful outcomes.[14] Earlier in history, Russian clinicians, in an attempt to achieve return of spontaneous circulation with patients experiencing cardiac arrest, snow was placed for cooling.[2] In the 1930s, victims rescued after asphyxiation from drowning in cold water proved successful resuscitation. With this finding came the idea from clinicians that subnormal temperatures provided neuroprotection against anoxic brain injury.[15] Investigators have tested with subnormal temperatures to protect the brain for more than 50 years. This was the idea for decreasing metabolic demand and oxygen consumption in the body.[16]

The first reported clinical application of hypothermia was performed by Fay in 1938. The procedure was limited to the terminally ill, who were subjected to temperatures of approximately 80°F (27°C). Hypothermia was used as a palliative care method for terminally ill patients with metastatic cancer for tumor shrinkage and pain relief. Also, his work continued on in neurosurgery and cardiothoracic surgery procedures, inducing deep hypothermia (15°C–22°C) for demonstrating an effective method of neuroprotection.[17]

Since the 1940s, numerous case reports and series and uncontrolled studies have reported possible benefits of induced hypothermia on neurologic outcome after cardiac arrest and traumatic brain injury (TBI). Many of these trials, however, were severely hindered by the side effects caused by cooling at subnormal temperatures. This made it challenging because patients were treated on general floors without the support of an ICU that could provide ventilatory and circulatory support. Furthermore, clinicians believed that body temperature needed to be at subnormal temperatures to achieve the benefits of decreased brain metabolism and oxygen demand. Between the dangerous side effects and mixed study results, large-scale acceptance of hypothermia as a medical method was disallowed, even though its use was practiced in the perioperative setting.[18]

During the mid-1980s and early 1990s, more laboratory studies using animal models were performed showing a clinical use of hypothermia. The data suggested that deep hypothermia was not needed to achieve the protective benefits that moderate to mild hypothermia (32°–35°C) could achieve with fewer harmful side effects. Also, the formation of ICUs has made it more possible to deal with the side effects of cooling.[18] A published guideline by Safar[19] in 1964 for heart and lung resuscitation recommended the induction of hypothermia if, within 30 minutes there was no sign of neurologic recovery. These early implementations did not turn into extensive clinical practice until 2002.[2]

IMPLICATIONS FOR TARGETED TEMPERATURE MANAGEMENT

The theory of intentional manipulation of patient temperature, also known as TTM, has come forth as a treatment method in critically ill neuroscience patients. The principal goal of TTM is to proactively inhibit the ill effects of fever by decreasing cerebral metabolism, stabilizing the blood-brain barrier, diminishing ischemic depolarization, and limiting free radial production so as to minimize or avert neuronal destruction and progression of secondary brain injury.[5,12]

Each patient's clinical condition and underlying disease process should drive eligibility for consideration of the therapy. No matter what the underlying disease process, patient temperature should be monitored frequently and infectious causes of fever should be pursued and treated. This article addresses caring for neurologically challenged patients in whom infectious causes have been appropriately addressed prior to initiation of TTM therapy.

CLINICAL APPLICATION OF TARGETED TEMPERATURE MANAGEMENT
Traumatic Brain Injury

TBI effects approximately 10 million people worldwide,[20] 2 million of whom are found in the United States, accounting for 300,000 TBI hospital admissions and 50,000 TBI-related mortalities and leaving 5 million TBI survivors with some form of disability.[21,22] Due to cultural changes, TBI will likely be placed as the leading cause of death and disability by 2020.[20] TBI causes both instantaneous and deferred injuries through physiologic, metabolic, and functional disorders. Consequences of poor outcomes lead to significant impact on patients, families, and society.

Spontaneous hypothermia on admission of a TBI patient has been found independently associated with poorer outcomes, possibly related in part to the correlation between hypothermia, coagulopathy, acidosis, extensive hypothalamic injury, and/or hypovolemic shock.[6,23] Further caution plays out in studies conducted against aggressive warming of hypothermic severe TBI patients in favor of a more controlled approach of rewarming at less than or equal to 0.25°C/h, because aggressive rewarming can invalidate any positive effects of intracranial pressure (ICP) control by causing a rebound systemic inflammatory response syndrome–like response characterized by vasodilation, hypotension, and rebound ICP elevations.[24,25]

A joint venture between the Brain Trauma Foundation, American Association of Neurological Surgeons, and Congress of Neurological Surgeons produced "Guidelines for Management of Severe Traumatic Brain Injury,"[26] which addressed induction of hypothermia as a management strategy in TBI patients. This collaborative effort could not provide for a strong recommendation for therapeutic hypothermia, instead suggesting that further investigation was required. Initial studies suggested promising outcomes related to induced hypothermia[27] but were unable to be replicated in further studies.[28,29] Some conflicting results were also presented, suggesting that mild hypothermia might improve outcomes at 3 months postinjury but also noted that another variable, prevention of hyperglycemia, might also be partly an explanation for these improved outcomes.[30] Many questions and concerns remain surrounding the concept of induced hypothermia and could serve as the basis for future research, such as identifying ideal core body temperature, outlining time frame for induction of therapy, describing duration of therapy, and delineating outcome measures and results.

On the opposite side of the spectrum, fever has been described in 68% of TBI patients within 72 hours of injury,[4,5] a timeframe making it less likely that hyperthermia can be credited to an infectious cause in favor of a central source.[31] Deviation from normothermia, either hypothermia or hyperthermia, in the TBI population is associated with higher morbidity and mortality.[32] The controversy, however, remains that some studies have challenged the claim that fever is detrimental in the TBI population, because fever triggers the immune system response by initiating the coagulation reaction and mobilizing infection fighting cells.[33] To summarize, contrasting findings have contributed to a dearth of evidence in guiding management of temperature in the TBI population (**Fig. 1**).

Elevated Intracranial Pressure/Intracranial Hypertension

The "Guidelines for Management of Severe Traumatic Brain Injury" provide for a level II recommendation that patients with severe TBI (Glasgow Coma Scale score 3–8 after resuscitation) and an abnormal CT of the head should have the benefit of ICP monitoring to best guide therapy, proactively aim to prevent secondary injury, and ultimately improve outcomes.[26]

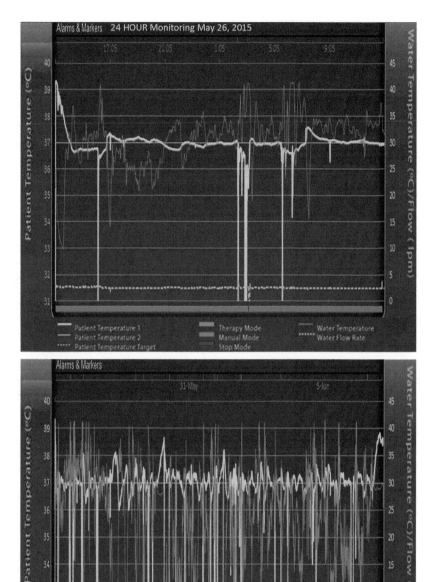

- Therapy started on 5/36 @ 13:05, patient temp 39.30°C.
- Target, 37°C, reached on 5/36 @ 14:10.
- The goal of normothermia was achieved within 1 hour of applying arctic sun pads and cooling.
- Overall temperature control was achieved throughout at the case.
- Total therapy time 308 hours and 7 minutes (13 days, 30 hours, and 7 minutes).
- The patient was following commands and discharged to an acute rehabilitation.

Fig. 1. Patient temperature in the TBI population. The blue semiconnected line on the bottom of the screen shows a continuous water flow representing that the machine is on and working. Sharp yellow drops of the patient's temperature during therapy correlate with probe movements that set off the alarms (this is represented on the top of the graphs with red markings). (*Courtesy of* Bard Medical Division, Covington, Georgia; with permission.)

In clinical practice, treatments targeted toward lowering ICP generally occur in a systemic stepwise fashion, beginning with positioning and then progressing toward more aggressive management. Although not well studied, interventions, such as targeting normotension, avoidance of hyperventilation or hypoventilation, avoidance of hypoxia, administration of osmotic diuretics, sedation/analgesia, cerebrospinal fluid diversion, and so forth, have few side effects. Similar to the discussion about usage of induced hypothermia and controlled normothermia in TBI patients, divergent opinions on utilization of TTM in severe TBI patients for treatment of intracranial hypertension can be found in the literature. ICP and cerebral perfusion pressure are known to be predictors of TBI outcomes, so randomization into groups that treat versus those that do not treat likely will not occur.

A systemic review was conducted by Sadaka and Veremakis (2012),[34] which described several studies that linked fever to intracranial hypertension and worsened outcomes. These investigators purport that induced hypothermia should be a consideration when more conventional measures have failed to control intracranial hypertension. The American Association of Neuroscience Nurses Clinical Practice Guidelines offer level 2 evidence (randomized controlled trial with important limitations) for maintaining normothermia as a proactive means of increased ICP increase control and induction of moderate hypothermia (33°C–36°C) as level 3 evidence (qualitative studies, case studies, clinical protocols, and expert opinion) in patients with refractory intracranial hypertension who did not receive barbiturates.[35] An additional concern is that of rebound intracranial hypertension during the rewarming process. It is essential that rebound increases in ICP be appropriately treated. Studies did not consistently show positive outcomes 6 months postinjury.

Ischemic Stroke

Approximately 795,000 people suffer from stroke each year in the United States, killing 129,000, thus placing stroke as the fifth leading cause of death in the United States as well as placing it as a leading cause of disability.[36]

A retrospective analysis of 110 ischemic stroke patients noted that temperatures (37.5°C–38°C) within the first 24 hours were associated with more severe symptoms,[5] whereas other investigators noted that febrile conditions occurred in more than 25% of ischemic stroke patients within the first 48 hours.[4] Clinical studies have suggested a strong independent link between temperature and stroke severity/outcomes. Biochemical activities that remain active for 3 to 5 days postinjury predispose patients to compromised penumbra and cerebral edema, leading to secondary injury.[37] The American Heart Association Scientific Statement, "Comprehensive Overview of Nursing and Interdisciplinary Care of the Ischemic Stroke Patient" (2009) maintain that normothermia (less than 37.6°C) should be the standard of care in stroke treatment with aggressive treatment of fever.[38–40]

Further exploration of the effects of temperature on ischemic strokes in animal models, noting that brain temperature is higher than body temperature, suggests that hypothermia might confine penumbral damage through limitation of infarct growth as well as restrict opening of the blood-brain barrier, thus diminishing cerebral swelling.[41]

Subarachnoid Hemorrhage

Temperature greater than 38.3°C has been reported in 72% of patients with subarachnoid hemorrhage (SAH), particularly within the first 10 days after SAH, with 50% having no infectious source.[4,5] Experimental animal models have established that blood within the cerebrospinal fluid pathway can induce fever, so the presence of intraventricular hemorrhage, poor Hunt-Hess grade and associated symptomatic cerebral vasospasm can be correlated with a strong threat for fever, which has been found independently associated with poor outcomes.[7,42,43] In addition, for every 1°C above 38.3°C, the odds mortality increases 22-fold.[44]

Similar to that of ischemic stroke, controlled normothermia lessens the burden of cerebral metabolism irrespective of elevated ICP.[45] A study conducted by Badjatia and colleagues (2010)[12] suggested that although limited by sample, maintenance of normothermia extended a patient's ICU stay and need for a tracheostomy but did not significantly seem to increase infectious complications and was beneficial toward outcomes.[12]

CONSIDERATIONS AND COMPLICATIONS

Induction of TTM can be accomplished through inexpensive and simple means, such as utilization of skin exposure to a cooled environment, ice packs in direct contact with skin, or infusion of cooled solutions. These interventions, although effective initial or short-term measures, can be labor demanding of nursing and do not allow for controlled maintenance or careful rewarming (especially in cases of induced hypothermia); however, they can still serve a purpose in the stepwise approach to temperature management.[18,25] Other considerations might include water circulating blankets or pads. Pharmacologic methods, such as acetaminophen (up to 4 g/24 h in absence of liver failure) serve as a useful adjunctive therapy when combined with environmental and evaporative interventions to decrease fever.[46]

Newer technology has facilitated more aggressive, tightly controlled temperature modulation through the use of both surface cooling with hydrogel pads and intravascular cooling devices. The hallmark of these devices is that they are driven by feedback mechanisms from a temperature probe (esophageal, rectal, bladder, and so forth) providing continuous input of temperature and attached to the device, which can automatically regulate temperature. Ability to trend the water temperature required to maintain a patient's temperature at a certain set point also provides additional data. If the water temperature is consistently low (indicating that the patient is trying to generate a fever, but the equipment is preventing a rise in temperature), further work-up might be indicated to rule out an infectious process.

One of the major adverse effects of controlling temperature, both induced hypothermia and even more so in controlled normothermia, is shivering. This untoward effect has been noted to affect approximately 64% of patients undergoing therapy.[18,47] During controlled normothermia, the body's counter-regulatory mechanisms within the hypothalamus attempts to conserve and generate heat at maximum efficiency.[18] Shivering is the result of skeletal muscular contraction and peripheral vasoconstriction used as a regulatory mechanism to increase heat production, by increasing metabolic rate, resting energy expenditure, oxygen uptake, and production of carbon dioxide. In theory, neuroprotection occurs by decreasing each 1°C, thereby decreasing the cerebral metabolic rate by 15%, so theoretically, shivering offsets any advantages of controlling temperature. An outcome of the 2011 Neurocritical Care Society's Multidisciplinary Consensus Conference on management of patients with an SAH was a strong recommendation made based on high-quality evidence that shivering should be monitored and controlled.[45] This can be generalized to most patients with underlying neuropathologies. Control of shivering is an essential adjuvant to maintaining both induced hypothermia and controlled normothermia.

Observational abilities by bedside practitioners allow for early detection of shivering and are the basis of the validated Bedside Shivering Assessment Scale (BSAS), which quantifies shivering (**Table 1**).[47] Using this 4-point scale based on palpation of neck,

Table 1		
Bedside Shivering Assessment Scale		
Score	Type of Shivering	Location
0	None	No shivering is detected on masseter, neck, or chest muscles
1	Mild	Shivering localized to neck and thorax only
2	Moderate	Shivering involves gross movement of upper extremities (in addition to the neck and thorax)
3	Severe	Shivering involves gross movement of trunk and upper and lower extremities

From Badjatia N, Strongilis E, Gordon E, et al. Metabolic impact of shivering during therapeutic temperature modulation: the bedside shivering assessment scale. Stroke 2008;39:3243; with permission.

masseter, chest muscles, and upper extremities is an objective assessment with 0 indicating no observation of shivering in any of the identified muscle groups; 1, mild shivering; 2, moderate shivering; and 3, severe neck, chest, and extremity shivering. Because this evaluation takes less than a minute to perform, it is easily incorporated into hourly vital signs. A BSAS of 2 or 3 is an indication for intervention to attain a goal of BSAS less than or equal to 1.

Approaches to shivering control should begin with the least aggressive, nonpharmacological actions and progress to more invasive interventions in a stepwise fashion. The use of noninvasive, nonsedating, and nonpharmacological interventions should be considered a beginning point for application of surface counterwarming to the hands and feet of patients, which is believed to counter the feedback loop from the skin temperature to the hypothalamic centers.[37] Young men with a lower body surface area seem at greatest risk of shivering.[48]

Several studies have proposed pharmacologic agents either used independently or in complement with others to reduce the body's thermoregulatory response to shivering.[25] These measures can be initiated prophylactically but almost always are continued for the duration of therapy. Oral medications, such as acetaminophen, are thought to lower the hypothalamic set point by acting by inhibiting cyclooxygenase-mediated prostaglandin synthesis. Buspirone, which is believed to act on serotonin type 1A to lower shivering threshold, can be considered a first-line pharmacologic intervention, as well as having a synergistic effect when used with other antishivering medications.[48]

Administration of parenteral opiates, such as meperidine and fentanyl, has advantages. Both medications possess analgesic properties, thereby also providing some level of pain control in addition to decreasing the shivering threshold. Meperidine lowers shivering threshold by its effects on α_{2B}-adrenoceptor subtypes, as much as twice that of other opioids, and complements both the effects of buspirone and dexmedetomidine.[49] Concern for its use is related to its many side effects, including lowering of the seizure threshold and respiratory depression.[48,50] Fentanyl, with its advantage of short action, likely reduces shivering in part due to its sedative properties but may also result in toxicities when used with hypothermia protocols.[50]

α-Agonists, such as dexmedetomidine, have secured a role in treatment of shivering, by acting on both vasoconstrictive and shivering thresholds. Although its clear advantage is related to the effects of decreased agitation with little risk of respiratory depression, concern for bradycardia (already a risk in induced hypothermia) may lead to hemodynamic instability.

Lower serum magnesium levels correlate with increases in shivering, so optimizing serum magnesium levels decreases shivering through what is thought to be vasodilation.[47,48,51] Benefits of magnesium infusions are its nonsedating effects coupled with the property of shortening time to goal temperature.[48]

Propofol used at higher levels (50–70 μg/kg/min) has sedative and amnesic properties, while mildly decreasing shivering and vasoconstrictive thresholds. Although some of these assets may position this medication in a desirable category, its use may be limited by hypotension, negative cardiac ionotropy, sedation, and potential for propofol infusion syndrome.[48]

Paralytics, although a highly effective short-term measure to terminate visible shivering, should be considered a last resort. The benefits of normotension with use is offset by significant disadvantages. When paralytics are used, the sensitive indicator of neurologic assessment is lost and clinically seizure activity cannot be observed. Another limiting factors is that visible signs of shivering abate; however, centrally, the brain continues to attempt to produce a shivering reaction; sedation still is required and the continued usage of paralytic agents increases risk of critical illness polyneuromyopathy.[18,48]

Although supported as a therapy in few neurologically impaired patients, induced hypothermia has the potential for additional complications, which can be mitigated by management of expert clinicians. These can include (but are not limited to) dysrhythmias, diminished left ventricular function, hypokalemia, hypotension, immunosuppression, suppression of inflammatory response possibly linked to increased infections, thrombocytopenia, mild coagulopathy (particularly if temperature is driven to <32°C), disruption to skin integrity due to vasoconstriction of vessels, insulin resistance/hyperglycemia, changes in drug clearances often due to slowing of liver enzymes, and hypovolemia secondary to diuresis due to a decrease in antidiuretic hormone (**Table 2**).[18,25,52]

Judicious, slow rewarming of the hypothermic patient, as well as an understanding of the process, is a proactive approach to prevention of complications. Comprehension of electrolyte shifts during rewarming, particularly with potassium moving intracellularly to extracellularly, helps practitioners avoid rapid rewarming, thus allowing the kidneys sufficient time to excrete excessive potassium.[18] Great care with rewarming should be taken with patients whose imaging reveals mass effect because the rewarming process can cause a rebound in ICP. If performed too rapidly, a rebound systemic inflammatory response syndrome–like response could be created characterized by vasodilation hypotension and rebound ICP. Significant imbalances in cerebrovascular activity can occur if patients are permitted to become hyperthermic after completing the rewarming process.[53]

Table 2
Potential complications of induced hypothermia

Cardiovascular	Immunologic	Hematologic	Metabolic	Miscellaneous
Dysrhythmias	Immunosuppression	Thrombocytopenia	Hypokalemia	Shivering
↓ Left ventricular function	↓ Inflammatory response	Mild coagulopathy	Hyperglycemia	Disruption to skin integrity
Hypotension	Leukopenia, impaired white blood cell migration, poor clearance of bacteremia			Changes in drug clearance/ elimination
				Hypovolemia

SUMMARY

There are many approaches and opportunities to implementing temperature modulation in critically ill patients, but barriers also exist. Conceptually, the process of cooling is straightforward; however, TTM is anything but simplistic. The need for a collaborative approach (physicians champions, nursing support, respiratory therapists, pharmacists, laboratory personnel, and supply chain representatives) to address definitions of normothermia and fever, patient inclusion/exclusion criteria for therapy based on underlying neurorelated pathologies, determination of methods of induction/maintenance, monitoring required, education planning, and strategies to minimize potential complications are warranted.

Unfortunately, although guidelines and recommendations support treatment of fever, the number of validated studies is insufficient; therefore, a recommendation can be offered to further explore opportunities. Currently, evidence-based standardized protocols are lacking; thus, initiation of treatment might be delayed by nurses' knowledge of fever management as well as individual physician orders.[10] This lack of knowledge results in decreasing efficiency in attaining target temperature. Bundled order sets and protocols decrease barriers, increase autonomy and empowerment, maintain a consistent approach, and improve communication among the team. Bedside clinicians have been placed in the distinctive situation of facilitating improved outcomes by addressing the need to treat fever.

REFERENCES

1. Peberdy MA, Callaway CW, Neumar RW, et al. Part 9: Post-cardiac arrest care: 2010 American Heart Association Guidelines for Cardiopulmonary Resuscitation and emergency cardiovascular care. Circulation 2010;122(18 Suppl 3):S768–86.
2. Perman SM, Goyal M, Neumar RW, et al. Clinical applications of targeted temperature management. Chest 2014;145(2):386–93.
3. Avery KR, O'Brien M, Pierce CD, et al. Use of a nursing checklist to facilitate implementation of therapeutic hypothermia after cardiac arrest. Crit Care Nurse 2015;35(1):29–38.
4. Mcilvoy L. Fever management in patients with brain injury. AACN Adv Crit Care 2012;23(2):204–11.
5. Beninga JG, Johnson KG, Mark DD. Normothermia for neuroprotection: It's hot to be cool. Nurs Clin North Am 2014;49(3):399–413.
6. Madden LK, DeVon HA. A systematic review of the effects of body temperature on outcome after adult traumatic brain injury. J Neurosci Nurs 2015;473(4): 190–213.
7. Badjatia N, Kowalski RG, Schmidt JM, et al. Predictors and clinical applications of shivering during therapeutic normothermia. Neurocrit Care 2007;6(3):186–91.
8. Ng L, Wang J, Altaweel L, et al. Neurologic aspects of cardiac emergencies. Crit Care Clin 2014;30(3):557–84.
9. Thompson HJ, Pinto-Martin J, Bullock MR. Neurogenic fever after traumatic brain injury: an epidemiological study. J Neurol Neurosurg Psychiatry 2003;74(5):614–9.
10. Rockett H, Thompson HJ, Blissitt PA. Fever management practices of neuroscience nurses: what has changed? J Neurosci Nurs 2015;47(2):66–75.
11. Kramer LW. Evidence based practice: fever evaluation and early recognition of systemic inflammatory response syndrome in critical care patients. Dimens Crit Care Nurs 2010;29(1):20–8.
12. Badjatia N. Fever control in the neuro-ICU: why, who and when. Curr Opin Crit Care 2009;15(2):79–82.

13. Greer DM, Funk SE, Reaven NL, et al. Impact of fever on outcome of patients with stroke and neurologic injury: a comprehensive meta-analysis. Stroke 2008; 39(11):3029–35.
14. Guly H. History of accidental hypothermia. Resuscitation 2011;82(1):122–5.
15. Faridar A, Bershad EM, Emiru T, et al. Therapeutic hypothermia in stroke and traumatic brain injury. Front Neurol 2011;80(2):1–11.
16. Clifton GL. Is keeping cool still hot: an update on hypothermia in brain injury. Curr Opin Crit Care 2004;10(2):116–9.
17. Harris OA, Colford JM Jr, Good MC, et al. The role of hypothermia in the management of severe brain injury: a meta-analysis. Arch Neurol 2002;59(7):1077–83.
18. Polderman KH. Induced hypothermia and fever control for prevention and treatment of neurologic injuries. Lancet 2008;371:1955–69.
19. Safar P. Community-wide cardiopulmonary resuscitation. J Iowa Med Soc 1964; 54:629–35.
20. Agoston DV. Bench-to-bedside and bedside back to the bench; seeking a better understanding of the acute pathophysiological process in severe traumatic brain injury. Front Neurol 2015;6:47.
21. Coronado VG, McGuire LC, Sarmiento K, et al. Trends in traumatic brain injury in the U.S. and the public health response. J Safety Res 2012;43(4):299–307.
22. Coronado VG, Xu L, Basavaraju SV, et al. Surveillance for traumatic brain injury-related deaths–United States, 1997-2007. MMWR Surveill Summ 2011;60(5):1–32.
23. Burkur M, Kurtovic S, Berry C, et al. Pre-hospital hypothermia is not associated with increased survival after traumatic brain injury. J Surg Res 2012;175(1):24–9.
24. Thompson HJ, Kirkness CJ, Mitchell PH. Hypothermia and rapid rewarming is associated with worse outcome following traumatic brain injury. J Trauma Nurs 2010;17(4):173–7.
25. Linhares G, Mayer SE. Hypothermia for the treatment of ischemic and hemorrhagic stroke. Crit Care Med 2009;37(7):S243–9.
26. Bratton S, Bullock MR, Carney N, et al. Guidelines for the management of severe traumatic brain injury. J Neurotrauma 2007;24(S1):S21–5.
27. Marion DW, Penrod LE, Kelsey SF, et al. Treatment of traumatic brain injury with moderate hypothermia. N Engl J Med 1997;336:540–6.
28. Clifton GL, Valadka A, Zygun D, et al. Very early hypothermia induction in patients with severe brain injury study: hypothermia II: a randomized trial. Lancet 2011; 10(2):131–9.
29. Tokutomi T, Miyagi T, Takeuchi Y, et al. Effect of 35° C hypothermia on intracranial pressure and clinical outcome in patients with severe traumatic brain injury. J Trauma 2009;66(1):166–73.
30. Zhao QJ, Zhang XG, Wang LX. Mild hypothermia therapy reduces blood glucose and lactate and improves neurologic outcomes in patients with severe traumatic brain injury. J Crit Care 2011;26(3):311–5.
31. Li J, Jiang J-Y. Chinese head trauma data bank: effect of hyperthermia on the outcome of acute head trauma patients. J Neurotrauma 2012;29(1):96–100.
32. Sacho RH, Vail A, Rainey T, et al. The effects of spontaneous alterations in brain temperature on outcome: a prospective observational cohort study in patients with severe traumatic brain injury. J Neurotrauma 2010;27(12):2157–64.
33. Laws C, Jallo J. Fever and infection in the neurosurgical intensive care unit. JHN J 2010;5(2):22–7. Available at: http://jdc.jefferson.edu/jhnk/vol5/iss2/5.
34. Sadaka F, Veremakis C. Therapeutic hypothermia for the management of intracranial hypertension in severe traumatic brain injury: a systemic review. Brain Inj 2012;26(7–8):899–908.

35. Mcilvoy L, Meyer K. Nursing management of adults with severe traumatic brain injury. AANN Clin Pract Guideline Ser 2012;1–20. Available at: http://www.aann.org. Accessed August 21, 2015.
36. American Heart Association. Heart and Stroke Statistics. Available at: http://www.heart.org/HEARTORG/General/Heart-and-Stroke-Association-Statistics_UCM_319064_SubHomePage.jsp. Accessed August 14, 2015.
37. Badjatia N, Strongilis E, Prescutti M, et al. Metabolic benefits of surface counter warming during therapeutic temperature modulation. Crit Care Med 2009;37(6):1893–7.
38. Thompson HJ. Evidence base for fever interventions following stroke. Stroke 2015;46:e98–100.
39. Summers D, Leonard A, Wentworth D, et al. Comprehensive overview of nursing and interdisciplinary care of the acute ischemic stroke patient. Stroke 2009;40:2911–44.
40. Aiyagari V, Diringer MN. Fever control and its impact on outcomes: what is the evidence? J Neurol Sci 2007;261(1–2):39–46.
41. Karaszewski B, Carpenter TK, Thomas RGR, et al. Relationships between brain and body temperature, clinical and imaging outcomes after ischemic stroke. J Cereb Blood Flow Metab 2013;33:1083–9.
42. Oddo M, Frangos S, Milby A, et al. Induced normothermia attenuates cerebral metabolic distress in patients with aneurysmal subarachnoid hemorrhage and refractory fever. Stroke 2009;40:1913–6.
43. Green DM, Burns JD, DeFusco CM. ICU management of aneurysmal subarachnoid hemorrhage. J Intensive Care Med 2013;28(6):341–54.
44. Fernandez A, Schmidt JM, Claasen J, et al. Fever after subarachnoid hemorrhage. Neurology 2007;68(13):1013–9.
45. Diringer MN, Bleck TP, Hemphill JC III, et al. Critical care management of patients following aneurysmal subarachnoid hemorrhage: recommendations from the neurocriticalcare society's multidisciplinary consensus conference. Neurocrit Care 2011;15:211–40.
46. Kasner SE, Wein T, Piriyawat P, et al. Acetaminophen for altering body temperature in acute stroke: a randomized clinical trial. Stroke 2002;33:130–5.
47. Badjatia N, Strongilis E, Gordon E, et al. Metabolic impact of shivering during therapeutic temperature modulation: the bedside shivering assessment scale. Stroke 2008;39:3242–7.
48. Choi AH, Ko SB, Presciutti M, et al. Prevention of shivering during therapeutic temperature modulation: the Columbia anti-shivering protocol. Neurocrit Care 2011;14:389–94.
49. Doufas AG, Lin CM, Suleman MI, et al. Dexmedetomidine and meperidine additively reduce the shivering threshold in humans. Stroke 2003;34(5):1218–23.
50. Liu-DeRyke X, Rhoney DH. Pharmacological management of therapeutic hypothermia-induced shivering. SCCM 2008. Available at: http://www.sccm.org/Communications/Critical-Connections/Archives/Pages/Pharmacological-Management-of-Therapeutic-Hypothermia-Induced-Shivering.aspx. Accessed August 13, 2015.
51. Zweifler RM, Voorhees ME, Mahmood M, et al. Magnesium sulfate increases the rate of hypothermia via surface cooling and improves comfort. Stroke 2004;35(10):2331–4.
52. Kupchik N. Development and implementation of a therapeutic hypothermia protocol. Crit Care Med 2009;37(7):S279–84.
53. Lavinio A, Timofeev I, Nortje J, et al. Cerebrovascular reactivity during hypothermia and rewarming. Br J Anaesth 2007;99:237–44.

Moving?

Make sure your subscription moves with you!

To notify us of your new address, find your **Clinics Account Number** (located on your mailing label above your name), and contact customer service at:

Email: journalscustomerservice-usa@elsevier.com

800-654-2452 (subscribers in the U.S. & Canada)
314-447-8871 (subscribers outside of the U.S. & Canada)

Fax number: 314-447-8029

Elsevier Health Sciences Division
Subscription Customer Service
3251 Riverport Lane
Maryland Heights, MO 63043

*To ensure uninterrupted delivery of your subscription, please notify us at least 4 weeks in advance of move.

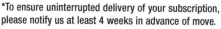

Printed and bound by CPI Group (UK) Ltd, Croydon, CR0 4YY

03/10/2024

01040491-0015